ASSESSMENT OF CELLULAR AND ORGAN FUNCTION AND DYSFUNCTION USING DIRECT AND DERIVED MRI METHODOLOGIES

Edited by **Christakis Constantinides**

Assessment of Cellular and Organ Function and Dysfunction using Direct and Derived MRI Methodologies
http://dx.doi.org/10.5772/61953
Edited by Christakis Constantinides

Contributors

David Moratal, Andrés Larroza, Vicent Bodí, Margaret Samyn, Kuo-Jung Lee, Eric Gottwald, Andreas Neubauer, Lothar Schad, Christakis Constantinides

Published by InTech

Janeza Trdine 9, 51000 Rijeka, Croatia

Publishing Process Manager Romina Rovan

Technical Editor SPi Global

Cover InTech Design team

First published October, 2016

Printed in Croatia

Additional hard copies can be obtained from orders@intechopen.com

Assessment of Cellular and Organ Function and Dysfunction using Direct and Derived MRI Methodologies , Edited by Christakis Constantinides

p. cm.

Print ISBN 978-953-51-2722-2
Online ISBN 978-953-51-2723-9

For EU product safety concerns:
IN TECH d.o.o., Prolaz Marije Krucifikse Kozulić 3, 51000 Rijeka, Croatia,
info@intechopen.com or visit our website at intechopen.com.

Meet the editor

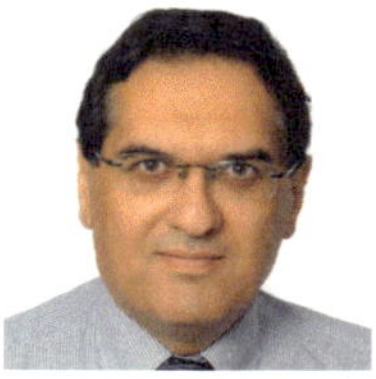

Christakis Constantinides completed his undergraduate studies at Imperial College London (BEngr., 1992) in Electrical/Electronic Engineering and his graduate and postgraduate studies at the Johns Hopkins University (MSc, 1994; PhD, 2000) in Biomedical Engineering. He has held appointments at NIH and as an assistant professor in the Department of Mechanical Engineering at the University of Cyprus (2005–2013). Currently he is a *Marie* Skłodowska-*Curie Fellow at the University of Oxford* (2015–2017). His research interests focus on cardiac function, tissue characterization, and cellular tracking methods using magnetic resonance imaging. He has published more than 80 papers in international peer-reviewed journals/conferences, 3 book chapters, and 3 books (2 of which as an editor). He serves as a reviewer for numerous high-impact journals and for ISMRM, EMBS, IEEE-SBI conferences, and EU's TDP Cost-Action.

Contents

Preface

Despite the tremendous growth in the field of magnetic resonance imaging (MRI) evidenced in the initial phases of its development in the early twentieth century, scientific focus has shifted in recent years toward the study of physiology and pathophysiology spanning the spatial scales of the molecule, cell, tissue, and organ. Intensified research activities over the past 15 years have justified efforts toward molecular and cellular imaging, dual-modality imaging systems, real-time acquisitions, dedicated image processing techniques and applications, and the critical evaluation of their potential translational value for use in the clinic. The integrative focus on molecular-cellular-tissue-organ function and dysfunction has taken a primary role in modern, personalized medicine, and it is envisaged to continue to do so, as accumulated knowledge from basic and clinical science work continues to elucidate molecular, cellular, and physiological/pathophysiological pathways and mechanisms.

In this scientific effort, MRI continues to play a critical and synergistic role from the perspectives of basic science, diagnosis, and clinical interventional/therapeutic approaches. Within the realm of the current role of MRI in modern medicine, this book summarizes state-of-the-art direct and derived MRI methodologies and approaches as applied toward the assessment of cellular and organ function and dysfunction. The contributions in this effort are not excessive but few, comprehensive, and distinguished and of high quality. The topic areas can be generalized to find applications in other scientific areas and span both brain and cardiac applications, extending interest to wider audiences.

The book opens with an Introductory Chapter in which Dr. Constantinides introduces and explains the nature and purpose of the book and the logic and significance of its contents.

In chapter 2, Dr. Neubauer and colleagues present a comprehensive and an analytical overview of the biophysical principles and fundamentals of MRI and nuclear magnetic resonance (NMR) techniques as these are applied to cellular functional studies, including applications that extend to metabolism and oxygen consumption, based on nuclei other than protons.

Professor Samyn and Dr. LaDisa in Chapter 3, introduce a novel and an interesting approach using MRI-based computational fluid dynamics (CFD) modeling to simulate and emulate the characteristics of flow, with applications to pediatric cardiovascular disease (acquired and congenital). The presented work is intriguing given its cross-discipline focus, a true manifestation of a successful collaborative effort that engages both engineers and clinicians.

In Chapter 4, Professor Lee extends novel state-of-the-art modeling MRI-derived approaches to functional brain activation through blood-oxygen-level-dependent mechanisms. The work uses a sparse generalized mixed-effect model to represent the spatial dependence of activated voxels and reduce dimensionality, thereby leading to computational benefits.

Of great interest is also the work presented in Chapter 5 by Dr. Larrozal and colleagues on the topic of texture analysis using MRI. The chapter is comprehensive and the overview emphasizes the increasingly important role of image processing in clinical diagnosis and medical practice. Given the cross-platform applicability of the presented work, I envisage that the chapter will stimulate increased interest from scientists and clinicians in a range of scientific disciplines.

Collectively, the book emphasizes quality work in thematic areas that span the spatial scales of the cell, tissue, and organ. I am hopeful that the book will serve to readers as a comprehensive reference guide of the current status and envisaged future direction of MRI in areas of basic science and clinical practice that are anticipated to have significant translational value.

With a great sense of humility and indebtedness, I would like to acknowledge InTech publications that have initiated and supported this effort to its completion.

Dr. Christakis Constantinides
Marie Skłodowska-Curie Research Fellow
Department of Cardiovascular Medicine
University of Oxford
Oxford, UK

Chapter 1

Introductory Chapter

Christakis Constantinides

Additional information is available at the end of the chapter

http://dx.doi.org/10.5772/65799

While early works on MRI focused on hardware and software developments, and the understanding of the biophysical principles, physiological, and pathophysiological phenomena that underlie MRI/NMR, in later years, efforts targeted improvements in acquisition speed, enhancement of image quality based on signal-to-noise-ratio benefits, multinuclear imaging, and the introduction of quantitative imaging/spectroscopy of metabolic, perfusion, and functional responses. Concerted parallel efforts targeted improvements in image quality through basic and advanced image processing techniques, capitalizing on advances in signal and digital image processing.

Scientific direction was strategically steered toward molecular imaging and personalized medicine in the early 2000, when focus groups at the National Institutes of Health (NIH) formulated scientific funding policies. Correspondingly, despite the inherent biophysical limitations of the phenomenon of NMR/MRI, the last 15 years have evidenced tremendous progress in breaking barriers toward molecular and intracellular imaging, synergistic or in competition with optical, positron-emission, and/or computer tomography.

In his chapter, Dr. Neubauer presents a succinct overview of the biophysical principles that govern spectroscopy and imaging of nuclei-other-than-protons, including sodium, potassium, and chlorine, and the ionic interactions with proteins. The chapter also extends to phosphorus and its value in the study of cellular metabolism and pH, and to the study of oxygen consumption. The study of ^{13}C techniques and novel MRI bioreactors are briefly introduced at the end of the chapter.

On the forefront of ^{1}H MRI, Drs. Samyn and LaDisa present an overview of computational fluid dynamics (CFD) modeling approaches based on MRI of large vessels. Phase contrast techniques were introduced in the late 1980s and early 1990s, work to study fluid flow, work among others that was independently pioneered by Drs. Dumoulin, Moran, Pelc, Firmin, and Mohiaddin. Tremendous advances have been documented ever since, especially for the study of large vessels, valvular disease, and cardiac chamber flow patterns. The high-resolution nature of ^{1}H MRI has allowed the construction of accurate anatomic 3D models that have been used in conjunction with computational flow dynamic techniques to provide accurate estimation of flow patterns in health and disease. Estimation of quantitative biomarkers, such as the wall shear stress, became successful through fluid-structure interaction modeling, ultimately dependent on material tissue properties and the constitutive law dependence. Such biomarkers became increasingly important since they correlated with inflammation and atherogenesis. Drs. Samyn and LaDisa present a comprehensive overview of CFD-based approaches for the estimation of WSS in cardiovascular disease (acquired and congenital), and the assessment of helical flow patterns and their benefits. More importantly, the discussion is extended to atherosclerosis in pediatric and in congenital heart disease.

In addition to cardiovascular disease, MR-based modeling has also been extensively applied in cerebrovascular applications, including functional MRI (fMRI). Dr. Lee introduces a Bayesian spatial-temporal model to capture the spatial dependence of brain-activated voxels. The sparsity of the proposed model leads to an increased computational efficiency. It is validated through a simulation and actual fMRI data paradigms.

Image processing has been integral to MRI since its inception. Texture analysis has emerged in the 1960s following the introduction of mathematical frameworks for non-orthogonal reconstruction schemes, including the wavelet algorithm. In the clinic, interest for texture analysis intensified in the early 1990s, particularly for breast cancer diagnosis. Dr. Larrozal and colleagues present a comprehensive overview of the progress of the field since its early days. The approach is modular and streamlined, and is presented in terms of the steps of MRI acquisition, regional image definition, pre-processing, feature extraction, and classification. The future evolution of this field targets clinical applicability, once reproducibility accuracy has been achieved, based on multicenter, international studies.

Collectively, in the effort to assess cellular and organ function and dysfunction using MRI-derived methodologies, the work presented in this book attests to the tremendous strides and accomplishments achieved thus far and projects to future directions aiming to attain translation in the clinic.

Author details

Christakis Constantinides

Address all correspondence to: christakis.constantinides@cardiov.ox.ac.uk

Department of Cardiovascular Medicine, University of Oxford, UK

Chapter 2

Tracking Cellular Functions by Exploiting the Paramagnetic Properties of X-Nuclei

Eric Gottwald, Andreas Neubauer and
Lothar R. Schad

Additional information is available at the end of the chapter

http://dx.doi.org/10.5772/64504

Abstract

The term X-nuclei summarises all nuclei (except protons) that occur in biological systems carrying a non-zero nuclear spin. Significant involvement in physiological processes such as maintaining the transmembrane potential of living cells and energy metabolism make these nuclei highly interesting for nuclear magnetic resonance (NMR) experiments. In this chapter, a discussion of the basic physics of nuclei with a nuclear spin >1/2 is presented. On this basis, pulse sequences for the detection of multi quantum coherences (MQCs) are presented and explained. Information contained in the obtained MQC signal is linked to biophysical processes. Applications to study energy metabolism, oxygen consumption, and to track brain metabolites by means of X-nuclei NMR are discussed as well as the use of functional phantoms, which can bridge the gap between basic biological research and NMR data interpretation.

Keywords: sodium, potassium, chlorine, functional phantoms, X-nuclei

1. Introduction

Apart from hydrogen (^{1}H) all nuclei carrying a non-zero nuclear spin can be used for signal generation in nuclear magnetic resonance (NMR), magnetic resonance imaging (MRI), and magnetic resonance spectroscopy (MRS) experiments. All these nuclei are referred to by the term *X-nuclei*. Sodium (^{23}Na) is the X-nucleus with the highest NMR sensitivity, and thus, it was already used for imaging 30 years ago [1]. In addition to ^{23}Na, there are other X-nuclei, which can be used for MRI/MRS experiments. Together with potassium (^{39}K), ^{23}Na mainly determines the cell membrane potential. Chlorine (^{35}Cl) is the most abundant anion in the human body, and its intracellular and extracellular concentrations have a huge impact on cell volume regulation. Oxygen (^{17}O) can give insight into the oxygen consumption of the tissue of interest. Phosphorus (^{31}P) is heavily involved in the energy metabolism (e.g. in skeletal muscle). Carbon (^{13}C) is the basis of all organic molecules and also enables the possibility to track brain metabolites. During the past years, several imaging techniques have been presented to exploit the signal of these nuclei [2].

The main question arising from the use of X-nuclei in MRI/MRS experiments is data interpretation. In biological systems, various processes are always occurring simultaneously, making it difficult to link a specific effect to an underlying physiological process. Therefore, methods are needed to bridge the gap between phantom experiments, which are used to develop new measurement techniques, and *in vivo* experiments. This can be accomplished with *functional phantoms* [3], which provide a high degree of control over biological processes, and therefore lead to a better understanding of the recorded signals.

This chapter gives an overview on the natural abundant X-nuclei, their physical properties, and physiological information, which can be obtained from NMR experiments with X-nuclei. Especially, the physics of X-nuclei with a nuclear spin >3/2 is discussed in detail with the goal to derive and understand enhanced pulse sequences for the observation of higher coherence orders. Applications for the spin 1/2 X-nuclei ^{17}O and ^{13}C are also discussed. The chapter closes with the introduction of a MRI compatible bioreactor setup, which can be used to study the response of organotypic cell cultures to external stimulations.

2. NMR sensitivity

Every nucleus used for NMR experiments has different physical properties and thus exhibits a different sensitivity response to radiofrequency (RF) pulses. The NMR sensitivity of a nucleus is given by:

$$S \propto C\gamma^3 I(I+1) \tag{1}$$

Here S is the sensitivity, C is the concentration of the nucleus, γ is the gyromagnetic ratio, and I represents the nuclear spin of the nucleus. Admittedly, most X-nuclei carry a nuclear spin > 1/2 which increases sensitivity. On the other hand, this effect is compensated by the much lower γ. Values for γ (relative to the value for ^1H), nuclear spin, natural abundances, and mean values of *in vivo* concentrations for the X-nuclei discussed here, are listed in **Table 1**. Since the nuclear spin and the gyromagnetic ratio are constants, the only variable in Eq. (1) is the concentration C. In contrast to ^1H, where the *in vivo* concentration reaches a molar (mol/l i.e. M) level, the concentrations of natural abundant X-nuclei is in the range of mM (mmol/l). For instance, ^{23}Na is the most abundant X-nucleus with the highest γ value but compared to ^1H the sensitivity is approximately 20,000 times lower.

Nucleus	Nuclear spin	Rel.γ	Natural abundance [%]	Mean *in vivo* concentration [mM]
^{1}H	1/2	1.00	99.98	88,000
^{13}C	1/2	0.25	1.11	n. a.
^{17}O	5/2	−0.14	0.037	16
^{23}Na	3/2	0.26	100.00	40
^{31}P	1/2	0.040	100.00	75
^{35}Cl	3/2	0.098	75.77	36
^{39}K	3/2	0.047	93.10	124

[1]Abundance in the whole body.

[2]Tissue ^{23}Na concentration in human brain.

[3]Tissue ^{35}Cl concentration in human brain.

[4]Concentration in human calf muscle. Since ^{13}C is mostly used for labelled precursors a value for *in vivo* concentration is lacking [4–8].

Table 1. Nuclear spin values, relative gyromagnetic ratios, natural abundances, and mean values of *in vivo* concentrations of different X-nuclei.

3. ^{23}Na, ^{35}Cl, and ^{39}K: interaction with proteins

The transmembrane potential mainly arises from concentration gradients of different ions between the intracellular and the extracellular compartments. Three X-nuclei, ^{23}Na, ^{35}Cl, and ^{39}K, and their intracellular/extracellular distribution play a major role in generating this potential. All three nuclei have a nuclear spin equal to 3/2, which leads to a nuclear quadrupolar moment Q and a fast decay of the NMR signal.

The nuclear quadrupolar moment is a measure of the deviation of the nuclear charge distribution from the spherical shape. Positive values of Q indicate, that the nuclear charge distribution takes the shape of a prolate spheroid while negative values indicate, that the nucleus takes the form of an inflate spheroid. The values for Q and the resulting shape of the discussed nuclei are listed in **Table 2**.

Nucleus	Quadrupolar moment Q [b]	Shape
^{17}O	−0.026*	Inflate spheroid
^{23}Na	+0.10*	Prolate spheroid
^{35}Cl	−0.10*,†	Inflate spheroid
^{39}K	+0.049*,†	Prolate spheroid

*Polarization or Sternheimer corrections incorporated.

†Average value [9].

Table 2. Quadrupolar moments and shapes of nuclei with nuclear spin >1/2.

The quadrupolar moment also implicates an additional electrical field which, in turn, leads to an additional contribution to the potential energy of the nucleus. This means that the energy levels, which split due to the Zeeman effect,[1] will be shifted due to the quadrupolar interaction, ω_Q, which is related to the electrical field induced by the quadrupolar moment. A description of the electrical field can be formulated using of the electrical field gradient (EFG) tensor, which can be found in references [10, 11]. **Figure 1** shows an illustration for the Zeeman effect in case of a spin 3/2 nucleus. On the left hand side of the figure, there is no external magnetic field and the energy levels are degenerate. Applying an external magnetic field nulls the degeneration and the energy levels split. In biological systems, the quadrupolar interaction can become time dependent. Therefore, it is useful to refer to the time averaged quadrupolar interaction $\langle\omega_Q\rangle$. For a non-zero external magnetic field and $\omega_Q = 0$, this is shown in the middle of **Figure 1**. The right hand side of **Figure 1** shows the case with an applied external magnetic field, where $\omega_Q \neq 0$. It can be seen that the inner transitions are shifted to lower energies while the outer transitions are shifted to higher energies. This leads to an alteration of the transition frequencies for the outer transitions.

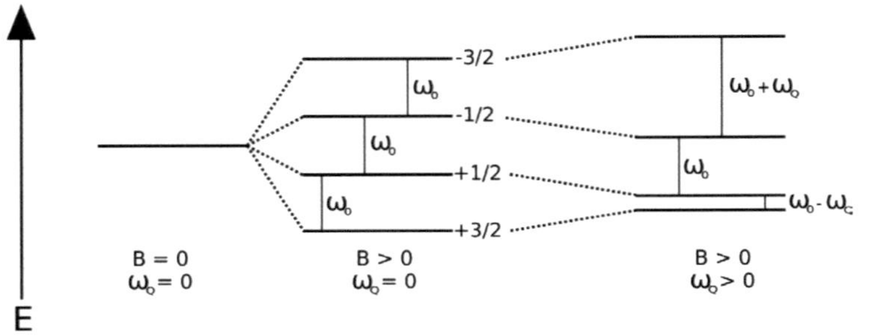

Figure 1. Zeeman effect in a spin 3/2 system. (Left) In the absence of an external magnetic field, the energy levels are degenerated. (Middle) Application of an external magnetic field leads (in the absence of a quadrupolar interaction) to an equidistant splitting of the energy levels. (Right) An additional quadrupolar interaction leads to a shift of the inner levels towards lower energy while the outer levels are shifted upwards. The end result is an alteration of the outer transitions.

The following paragraphs contain the description of the physical properties of signal generation and relaxation these nuclei. From this basis, dedicated pulse sequences for the observation of *multi quantum coherences* (MQCs) are derived. Applications of these sequences to phantoms are shown while the obtained data are analysed with the link to a physiological interpretation.

3.1. Quadrupolar relaxation

This section deals with the specific relaxation processes of quadrupolar nuclei. The detailed understanding of these processes requires a strong background in quantum physics, and the use of the irreducible tensor formalism which is beyond the scope of this book. For this reason, only the key results of the quantum mechanical description are presented in this chapter. The reader can find a more detailed description in references [10–12].

Taking this into account one can deduce the following two respective expressions for the real and imaginary parts (J_m and K_m) of the spectral density [11]:

$$J_m(m\omega_0) = \frac{(2\pi)^2}{20} \frac{\chi^2 \tau_c}{1 + (m\omega_0 \tau_c)^2} \quad (2)$$

$$K_m(m\omega_0) = \omega_0 \tau J_m(m\omega_0) \quad (3)$$

In the latter equations, ω_0 is the resonance frequency, τ is the length of the excitation pulse, τ_c is the rotational correlation time, which is a measurement for the degree of freedom of a nucleus, χ represents the root mean square coupling constant, and m is an integer number, which will be discussed later. Since no other correlation time will be discussed in this chapter, the rotational correlation time will be referred only as correlation time.

If nuclei can move freely, like in isotropic liquids, the correlation time is rather small and in the range of ns. If the motion becomes more restricted, like it is the case during the interaction with macromolecules, such as proteins, the correlation time increases. The quadrupolar coupling constant ω_Q is accounted for in the spectral density via the parameter χ. In biological systems, there is an increased variability of different environments and simultaneously ongoing processes leading to local variations of ω_Q, which justifies the usage of the root mean square value χ.

The influence of τ_c and ω_Q on the spectral density was extensively discussed by Rooney et al. [13]. In their paper, they defined four different regimes for τ_c and ω_Q resulting in four different types of spectra which are shown in **Figure 2**. These four regimes are:

- *Type a spectrum:* $\omega_Q \tau_c \gg 1$ and $\omega_0 \tau_c \gg 1$ and an additional macroscopic anisotropy in the sample (e.g. single or liquid crystals). Molecular motion is hardly present in this system which leads to distinct energy levels and three very narrow resonances comprising the central resonance and two symmetrical satellite resonances at higher and lower frequencies, respectively

- *Type b spectrum:* $\omega_Q \tau_c \gg 1$ and $\omega_0 \tau_c \gg 1$ and a random distribution of the orientation of the EFG tensors (e.g. inhomogeneous powder). Similar to the case of type a, molecular motion is hardly present but the random distribution of the EFG tensors leads to a broadening of the energy levels. In contrast to type a, where the spectrum shows three sharp lines, the satellite transitions become broadened due to many different values for ω_Q, and form a powder spectrum

- *Type c spectrum:* $\omega_Q \tau_c \ll 1$ and $\omega_0 \tau_c > 1$ and restricted motion (e.g. due to the interaction with proteins). In this type, the molecular motion is much higher than in the latter two. As a result, the energy levels are continually modulated and the satellite transitions vanish. As it can be seen (second column from the left) in **Figure 2** , the satellite resonances are completely vanished and the central resonance takes the shape of a Lorentzian which is also influenced by the orientation of the different EFG tensor orientations with respect to the external magnetic field (super-Lorentzian)

- *Type d spectrum:* $\langle\omega_Q\rangle = 0$ and $\omega_0\tau_c \ll 1$. This is the case in isotropic liquids. Due to rapid molecular motion, the time average of the quadrupolar interaction vanishes and the energy levels become sharp again. Moreover, there is no difference between the different transitions leading to a single, sharp resonance at ω_0

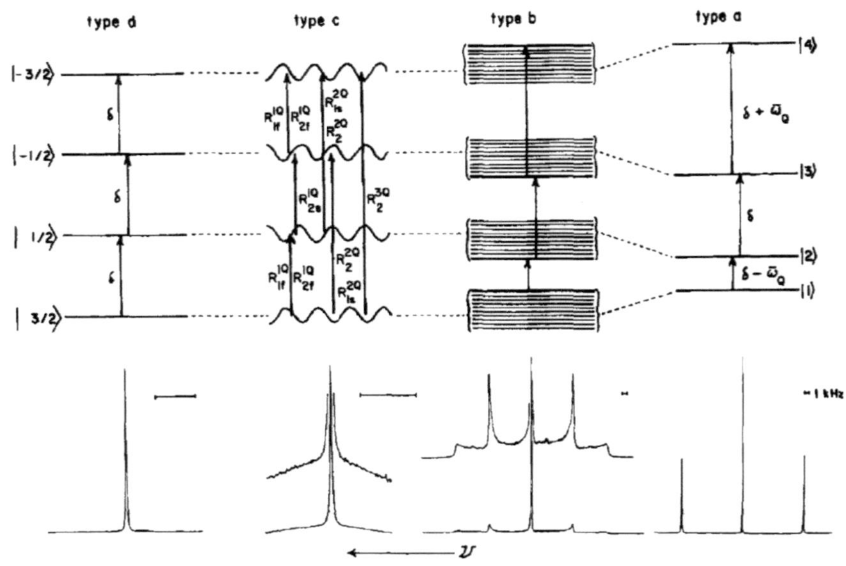

Figure 2. The four possible regimes for ^{23}Na spectra according to Rooney et al. Figure drawn from reference [13]. Copyright permission by John Wiley & Sons Ltd (license no. 3824201099423).

As it can be seen in **Figure 2**, nuclei with a nuclear spin > 1/2 can exhibit more than just one resonance. Therefore, transitions equal multiple times of the resonance frequency are possible. These transitions are known as *multi quantum coherences (MQCs)*. In the case of spin 3/2 nuclei, single quantum (SQ) coherences can be observed, which are normally used for proton MRI and two MQCs, double quantum (DQ) coherences and triple quantum (TQ) coherences, respectively. In order to understand the relaxation properties of SQ coherences, a homogeneous and isotropic environment with only one compartment is assumed. The detailed discussion of higher coherences will be treated separately.

3.1.1. Longitudinal relaxation

As known from ^{1}H-NMR the specific time constant T_1 for the longitudinal relaxation can be determined by usage of an inversion recovery (IR) sequence. After an initial 180° pulse follows an evolution period called inversion time (T_i). Observable magnetization is then generated by an additional 90° excitation pulse.

If the time between the last pulse and the acquisition is kept minimal, the acquired signal can be formulated according to reference [11]:

$$S(S_0,T_i) = S_0\left(1-\frac{2}{5}\left(e^{-R_1^0 T_i} + 4e^{-R_2^0 T_i}\right)\right) \tag{4}$$

with S_0, the signal which can be obtained in the case $T_i = 0$, and with the relaxation rates

$$R_1^0 = 2J_1 \tag{5}$$

$$R_2^0 = 2J_2 \tag{6}$$

While the relaxation rates R_1^0 and R_2^0 are given by the spectral densities J_1 and J_2 [11]:

$$J_1 = \frac{(2\pi)^2}{20}\frac{\chi^2\tau_c}{1+(\omega_0\tau_c)^2} \tag{7}$$

$$J_2 = \frac{(2\pi)^2}{20}\frac{\chi^2\tau_c}{1+(2\omega_0\tau_c)^2} \tag{8}$$

Here, it should be pointed out that the integer m, which was mentioned in the definition of the spectral densities (see Eqs. (2) and (3)), takes the values of 1 and 2. Theoretically, a biexponential relaxation curve which contains a fast and a slow relaxing component can be observed. However, it is very difficult to observe a biexponential T_1 relaxation, especially in biological tissue. Nevertheless, for ^{35}Cl a biexponential T_1 relaxation has been observed *in vivo* [14, 15].

It is common to express the relaxation rates with their inverse value, which leads to two different time constants:

$$T_{1f} = \frac{1}{R_1^0} \tag{9}$$

$$T_{1s} = \frac{1}{R_2^0} \tag{10}$$

T_{1f} depicts the time constant for the fast, and T_{1s} for the slow relaxing component. In the extreme narrowing limit $\omega_0\tau_c \ll 1$ (i.e. isotropic liquid), it follows that $T_{1f} = T_{1s}$. Therefore, the relaxation becomes monoexponential with the time constant T_1 and the signal equation simplifies to

$$S(S_0, T_i) = S_0\left(1 - 2e^{\frac{-T_i}{T_1}}\right) \tag{11}$$

3.1.2. Transverse relaxation

To measure the characteristic time constant T_2 for the longitudinal relaxation, spin echo (SE) sequences are commonly used. These sequences begin with an initial 90° excitation pulse. Subsequent to this pulse a 180° inversion pulse is placed in the middle of an evolution interval called echo time (T_E).

A more detailed version of the following description for the elicited SE signal can be found in reference [11]. The SE signal takes the form:

$$S(S_0, T_E) = S_0\frac{1}{5}\left(3e^{-R_1^1 T_E} + 2e^{-R_2^1 T_E}\right) \tag{12}$$

S_0 is the signal intensity when T_E is minimal and the relaxation rates are represented by:

$$R_1^1 = J_0 + J_1 \tag{13}$$

$$R_2^1 = J_1 + J_2 \tag{14}$$

In this case, the spectral density with m = 0 equals

$$J_0 = \frac{(2\pi)^2}{20}\chi^2\tau_c \tag{15}$$

where J_1 and J_2 are the same spectral densities defined in Eqs. (7) and (8). Expressing the relaxation rates with their inverse and leads to

$$T_{2f} = \frac{1}{R_1^1} \tag{16}$$

$$T_{2s} = \frac{1}{R_2^1} \tag{17}$$

Similar to the case of T_1 relaxation, the T_2 relaxation is biexponential and consists of a fast relaxing component with relaxation time T_{2f} and a slow relaxing component with a relaxation time T_{2s}. In the extreme narrowing limit, the relaxation times become equal and lead to a monoexponential relaxation. In contrast to longitudinal relaxation, the two components of the transverse relaxation can be measured straight forward. Examples can be found in references [14, 15].

3.1.3. Rotational correlation time and its influence on relaxation times

As referred to in the discussion of longitudinal and transverse relaxation time, the rotational correlation time τ_c, and the root mean square value of the quadrupolar interaction constant χ appear in each of these two processes. The relaxation rates of longitudinal and transverse relaxation can be used to determine τ_c and χ in a model with a single compartment. However, since the biexponential behaviour can be observed much easier in transverse relaxation, the relaxation rates R_1^1 and R_2^1 are used here to determine τ_c and χ. Additionally, the substitution $x = (\omega_0 \tau_c)^2$ is used.

First, the ratio a_1 of the two relaxation rates can be calculated as

$$a_1 = \frac{R_1^1}{R_2^1} = \frac{(2+x)(1+4x)}{2+5x} \tag{18}$$

Rearranging Eq. (18) for τ_c leads to:

$$\tau_c = \frac{1}{\omega_0} \sqrt{\frac{-9+5a_1 \pm \sqrt{25a_1^2 - 58a_1 + 49}}{8}} \tag{19}$$

Knowledge of τ_c can then be used to calculate the value for χ. Herein, the first step is to compute the difference b_1 of the relaxation rates:

$$b_1 = R_1^1 - R_2^1 = \frac{4\pi^2}{5} \chi^2 \tau_c \frac{x}{1+4x} \tag{20}$$

Solving for χ leads to,

$$\chi = \frac{1}{2\pi}\sqrt{\frac{5b_1(1+4x)}{\tau_c x}} \tag{21}$$

In order to study the behaviour of the relaxation times under the influence of τ_c, a constant value for χ is assumed. From Eq. (19) follows that τ_c depends on the resonance frequency and thus on the magnetic field strength, leading to a dependence of all relaxation times on the magnetic field strength. **Figure 3** shows the simulated behaviour of the product of T_1 and T_2 with χ being dependent on τ_c for magnetic field strengths of 9.4 T and 21.1 T. For the longitudinal relaxation, the assumed monoexponential behaviour leads to a single longitudinal relaxation time constant T_1. In case of the transverse relaxation, a biexponential behaviour was assumed, which leads to a fast relaxing (T_{2f}) and a slow relaxing (T_{2s}) component of the transverse relaxation time constant T_2. The value for τ_c, where the product $\omega_0\tau_c = 1$, is indicated with the dotted red lines for both field strengths. At increasing correlation times, it can be clearly seen that the fast transverse relaxation time is continuously decreasing. Time constants for longitudinal relaxation as well as the constants for slow transverse relaxation first decrease at an increasing correlation time. Around the area $\omega_0\tau_c = 1$, the relaxation times start to increase again. This clarifies why the value for longitudinal relaxation times in solids is of the order of seconds, whereas it is in the range of milliseconds for liquids.

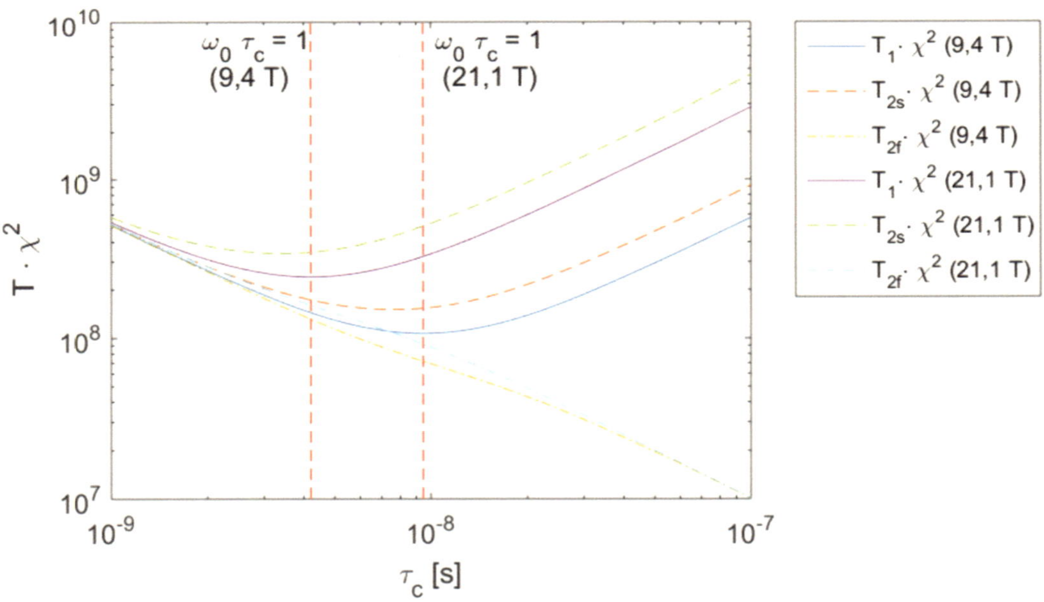

Figure 3. Dependence of relaxation times on the correlation time. Longitudinal as well as the slow components of transverse relaxation times initially decrease at increasing correlation times. Above the extreme narrowing limit, these relaxation times increase again. Short components of transverse relaxation times fall continuously at increasing correlation times.

3.1.4. Multi quantum coherences

As mentioned earlier, X-nuclei with a nuclear spin > 1/2 can exhibit MQCs. The theoretical description of MQCs is very complex and requires a background in quantum mechanics, a formulation that is outside the scope of this book. However, very extensive descriptions can be found in references [11, 16, 17].

MQCs can be a valuable tool for providing physiological information in MRI experiments. X-nuclei such as ^{23}Na, ^{35}Cl, and ^{39}K, which are heavily involved in physiological processes possess a nuclear spin equal to 3/2, and can therefore be used to generate MQCs. **Figure 4** shows all possible coherences in a spin 3/2 system. SQ and DQ coherences can be found in liquids as well as in environments with restricted motion. The most specific coherence is the TQ coherence. This coherence can only be found above the extreme narrowing limit $\omega_0 \tau_c \geq 1$, which can only be reached when there is at least temporary binding. In biological systems, this is realized by the interaction with macromolecules, such as proteins. For that reason, the intensity of the TQ signal can give insight in the amount of interaction between ions and proteins. Therefore, the sequences presented subsequently, exclusively deal with the generation and detection of SQ and TQ coherences.

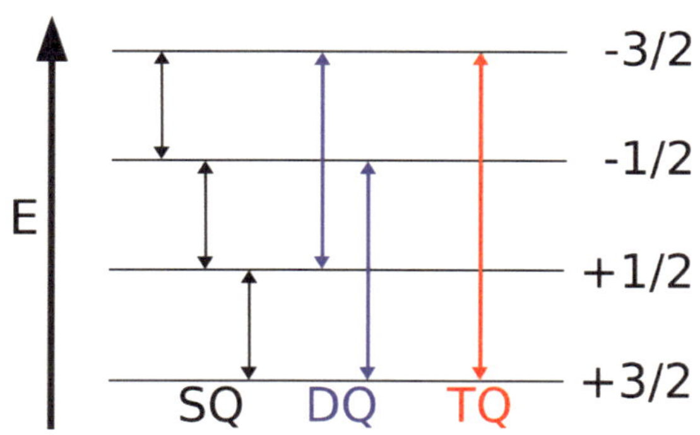

Figure 4. Multi quantum coherences in a spin 3/2 system. (Black) single quantum (SQ) transitions occur between neighbouring levels. (Blue) Double quantum (DQ) transitions skip one energy level. (Red) triple quantum (TQ) transitions skip two energy levels.

If pulsed excitation is used, like in common NMR spectrometers or MRI scanners, it is not possible to record MCQs directly. Instead of direct excitation with a single RF pulse, several excitation pulses need to be applied to generate a signal which includes MCQs. Typically, the signal generated by MCQs is much weaker than signal generated SQ coherences. As a result, one has to apply filter techniques to suppress contributions from unwanted coherences. There are two ways to filter different coherences: either through the application of gradient pulses, or by cycling the phases of applied pulses and/or the receiver.

Usage of gradient pulses is associated with the advantage of short total measurement times but the signal intensity is reduced by a factor of two. If phase cycling is used, the sequence must be repeated several times, each time with a different set of pulses and/or receiver phases.

If one deals with TQ coherences, the avoidance of signal loss is often more important than saving scanning time. For this reason, phase cycling is the preferred method in this chapter. Nevertheless, the reader can find some examples for filtration with gradient pulses in reference [18].

A common method for exciting and detecting TQ coherences is a pulse scheme consisting of three 90° excitation pulses, as illustrated in **Figure 5**. As it can be seen, all pulses have the same amplitude, while the phases of the first two pulses can vary. The time period between the first and the second pulse is called evolution time τ_{Evo}, and it is typically within the range of ms. Between the second and the third pulse, there is another short delay called mixing time, τ_{Mix}, which is typically in the range of several μs. In the case of TQ filtration, Φ' is set to 90° while Φ is cycled through the values of 30°, 90°, 150°, 210°, 270°and 330°. In addition to this, the receiver phase is altered between 0° and 180° after each subsequent scan and the phase of the third pulse is constantly equal to 0°. During the second pulse of the phase cycle, each coherence will accumulate the phases linearly, according to the number of energy levels which where skipped, i.e. DQ coherences will accumulate the phase with a factor one, and TQ coherences with a factor of two, respectively. In the literature, this is referred to as *triple quantum filtered* T_2 *(TQF-*T_2*)* experiment, or simply, a TQF experiment.

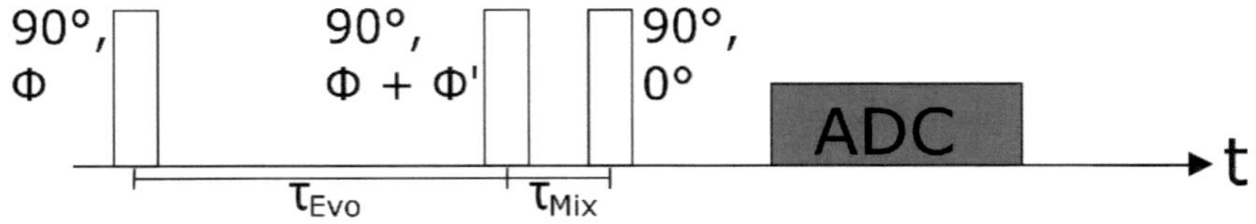

Figure 5. Three-pulse scheme for excitation and detection of MCQs. Pulse phases are indicated with Φ and Φ'. The time delays τ_{Evo} and τ_{Mix} represent evolution and mixing time. Data acquisition is indicated with ADC which refers to the analogue-to-digital converter.

The actual signal is obtained by complex addition of all subsequent scans. **Table 3** shows the phases accumulated by all coherences during the TQF experiment. As it can be seen from the values listed in **Table 3**, the contribution from SQ and DQ coherences cancel each other out while the phases of the TQ contributions are constant. After addition, the TQ signal can be expressed with the following equation [11]:

$$S(\tau_{Evo}) = \frac{15}{16}\frac{\sqrt{6}}{5}\left(e^{-R_1^1\tau_{Evo}} - e^{-R_2^1\tau_{Evo}}\right) \tag{22}$$

The relaxation rates R_1^1 and R_2^1 were defined in Eqs. (13) and (14). To avoid the influence of the acquisition time of the generated free induction decay (FID), a Fourier transform (FT) can be performed along the acquisition time domain. The dependence of τ_{Evo} is then found at ω_0 along the direction of τ_{Evo}.

SQ	DQ	TQ
30°	150°	270°
90°	90°	270°
150°	30°	270°
210°	330°	270°
270°	270°	270°
330°	210°	270°

Table 3. Accumulated phases of the different coherences during the TQF experiment.

Situations with $\omega_0\tau_c \geq 1$ can be easily simulated using solutions and the addition of agarose. The more agarose the sample contains, the higher the correlation time. In order to simulate different *in vivo* situations the agarose concentration can be varied from 1 to 7.5%. From this data, the correlation time can be extracted according to the one compartment model. This phantom data can help to interpret *in vivo* data regarding to the degree of ion binding. **Figure 6** shows the TQF signals of ^{23}Na in samples with different agarose concentration and 154 mM ^{23}Na concentration in dependence of the evolution time τ_{Evo} recorded at 9.4 T. All curves were normalized after acquisition and fitted according to the signal equation. With increasing agarose levels, one can clearly see an increase in the *signal-to-noise ratio (SNR)* indicating that the interaction of the ^{23}Na ions with their environment is also increasing. Additionally, the curves exhibit faster rise and decay times with increasing agarose, which is equivalent to an increase in both relaxation rates and a decrease in both relaxation times, respectively.

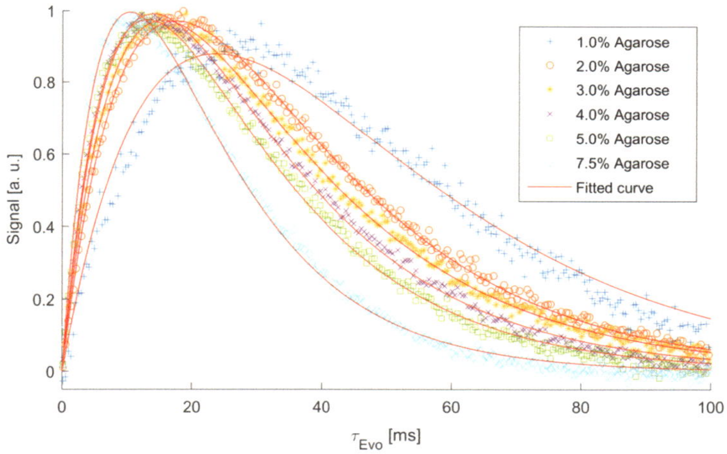

Figure 6. TQF signal of ^{23}Na at different agarose concentrations as a function of τ_{Evo} at 9.4 T. Increasing agarose content leads to an increased interaction between ^{23}Na and its environment, therefore, the TQF signal also increases. Additionally, both relaxation times become shorter, leading to a more rapid rise and decay of the signal.

As previously mentioned, the degree of binding will lead to an increase in TQ contributions.

If one wants to record dynamic processes, such as changes in the amount of free water or ion concentrations, a reference is needed. In *in vivo* experiments, it is often difficult to work with an external reference which underlies variations in transmit and receive fields. It would be more accurate to generate a spectrum with an intrinsic reference. In case of ^{1}H-MRS or ^{31}P-MRS, a spectrum with multiple peaks arises from different binding partners of the nucleus under observation. Unfortunately, X-nuclei with nuclear spin > 1/2 hardly have permanent binding partners. In most cases, the binding is related to interactions with macromolecules and cannot be seen in conventional spectroscopy.

SQ	DQ	TQ
90°	270°	90°
90°	90°	90°
135°	0°	225°
135°	180°	225°
180°	90°	0°
180°	270°	0°
225°	180°	135°
225°	0°	135°
270°	270°	270°
270°	90°	270°
315°	0°	45°
315°	180°	45°
0°	90°	180°
0°	270°	180°
45°	180°	315°
45°	0°	315°

Table 4. Phases of different coherences by applying triple quantum filtered time proportional phase increment (TQTPPI) spectroscopy with DQ suppression.

The solution to this problem is provided by multi quantum (MQ) spectroscopy. A very promising sequence to generate more resonance peaks from different MQCs in a single spectrum is referred to with the term *triple quantum filtered time proportional phase increment (TQTPPI)* [19]. The sequence diagram is basically the same shown in **Figure 5**. The only difference is the applied phase cycle and the fact that τ_{Evo} is incremented after each step in the phase cycle. Since DQ coherences also occur in liquids, a suppression of these contributions can help to simplify the signal and can be achieved by application of a 16 step phase cycle starting with $\Phi = 90°$, for the first pulse. The second pulse carries the variable phase Φ and the constant phase $\Phi' = 90°$ and the phase of the third pulse is, like the receiver phase, equal to zero. In order to suppress DQ coherences, each step in the phase cycle has to be repeated twice, the second time with an additional 180° phase on the middle pulse. Incrementing Φ and τ_{Evo} is then performed after each second step in the phase cycle. Typical values for Φ and τ_{Evo} are 45° and 100μs. **Table 4** shows the resulting phases of all occurring coherences after application of the 16 step phase cycle. It can be seen that in the case of SQ and TQ contributions, the phases of two subsequent scans are equal, while the two subsequent phases for DQ contributions differ by 180°. DQ suppression can then be achieved by the addition of the two subsequent scans.

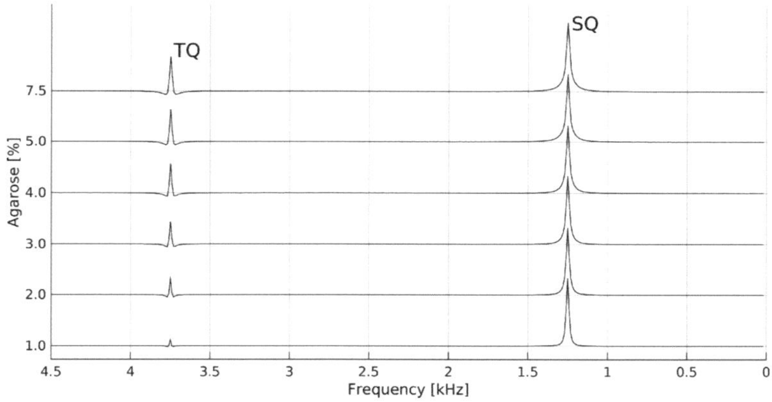

Figure 7. TQTPPI spectra of ^{23}Na at 9.4 T with different concentrations of agarose. The frequency increases from right to left. All curves were normalized with respect to the SQ resonance. At increasing agarose content (shown along the y-axis), the TQ contribution becomes more pronounced.

Generating the desired signal includes two steps: First, a FT has to be performed in the acquisition domain. Second, a second FID is generated by taking the points at ω_0 in the evolution time domain. This second dimension FID can be therefore turned into a spectrum by the application of an additional FT. Only the experimental results of this sequence are shown. Interested readers can find a very detailed derivation of the signal equation in reference [17].

Figure 7 shows TQTPPI spectra with DQ suppression of ^{23}Na obtained at 9.4 T. Different agarose concentrations are located along the y-axis. The first peak from the right is the SQ resonance which is located at 1.25 kHz. Accordingly, the TQ resonance appears at a frequency of 3.75 kHz which is exactly three times the SQ frequency. All of the spectra are normalized to the maximum value of the SQ resonance. One can clearly see the gain in TQ signal at increasing agarose concentrations. It is possible to consider the SQ peak as an internal reference, to calculate the area under both peaks and to build the ratio TQ/SQ. Observing the TQ/SQ ratio allows the conduct of dynamic studies of changes in the motional freedom induced by changes in the binding of the nucleus under investigation. If applied to biological tissue, this can give valuable information about the amount of bound ions and their interaction with proteins in the tissue.

3.2. ^{31}P: Energy metabolism

^{31}P spectroscopy has found its way into basic and clinical research due to the fact that ^{31}P is involved in energy metabolism. Energy consuming processes, such as the maintenance of the membrane potential, use the hydrolysis of adenosine triphosphate (ATP) as the energy source. The reaction is in accordance to:

$$ATP + H_2O \rightarrow ADP + P_i \tag{23}$$

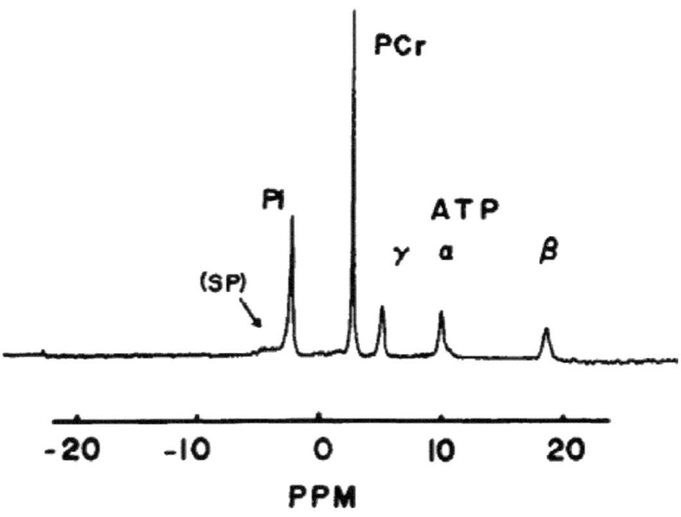

Figure 8. ^{31}P spectrum of a resting, arterially perfused cat soleus muscle. One can clearly see the phosphocreatine (PCr) resonance. The α, β, and γ resonances of adenosine triphosphate (ATP) are found at positive values for δ, while the inorganic phosphate (Pi) resonates at negative δ values. Contributions of sugar phosphate (SP) are also found at negative δ values. Figure drawn from reference [20]. Copyright permission by The American Physiological Society (license no. 3871910770507).

It can be seen that adenosine diphosphate (ADP) and inorganic phosphate (Pi) are produced during this reaction. In addition to the resonances of ATP, ADP and Pi one can also detect ^{31}P resonances from phosphomonoesters and diesters. **Figure 8** shows an example for a ^{31}P spectrum recorded from a resting, arterially perfused cat soleus muscle [20]. One can clearly see the three resonances of ATP, the phosphocreatine (PCr) resonance, and the resonance line of Pi. Small contributions from sugar phosphate (SG) are also visible.

http://dx.doi.org/10.5772/64504

An overview of resonances of detectable metabolites is shown in **Table 5** [4]. As it can be seen from **Table 5**, the chemical shift (δ) of the different metabolites covers a wide range. By convention, the PCr resonance is set as internal reference ($\delta = 0.00$ ppm).

Metabolite	Chemical shift
Adenosine monophosphate (AMP)	6.33
Adenosine diphosphate (ADP)	-7.05 (α)
	-3.09 (β)
Adenosine triphosphate	-7.52 (α)
	-16.26 (β)
	-2.48 (γ)
Dihydroxyacetone phosphate	7.56
Glucose-1-phosphate	5.15
Glucose-6-phosphate	7.20
Inorganic phosphate (P_i)	5.02
Phosphocreatine (PCr)	0.00
Phosphoenolpyruvate	2.06
Phosphoryl choline	5.88
Phosphoryl ethanolamine	6.78
Nicotinamide adenine dinucleotide (NADH)	-8.30

Table 5. Detectable metabolites by ^{31}P spectroscopy with their chemical shift.

In ^{31}P applications, it is not only possible to measure the concentration of a metabolite, it is also possible to derive rate constants based on changes of the concentrations of the PCr, Pi, and ATP. To influence the concentrations of PCr, Pi, and ATP, it is common to acquire the data while a volunteer is exercising and during the recovery period after the exercise. In the literature, one can find a variety of studies of the energy metabolism of human calf muscles. An extensive review is presented in reference [21].

The fact that the chemical shift of many ^{31}P resonances is dependent on the intracellular pH and magnesium concentration, leads to another interesting application, namely, the *in vivo* measurement of pH values. This can be achieved using the Henderson-Hasselbach equation:

$$pH = pK + log\left(\frac{\delta - \delta_{HA}}{\delta_A - \delta}\right) \tag{24}$$

where pK is the equilibrium constant for the acid-base equilibrium between A and HA. The chemical shifts of the protonated and dissociated forms of the molecule under observation are expressed by δ_{HA} and δ_A, respectively. Determining pH is achieved by measuring the chemical shift δ between PCr and Pi. With literature values, Eq. (24) takes the form [22]:

$$pH = 6.803 + log\left(\frac{\delta - 3.22}{5.73 - \delta}\right) \tag{25}$$

3.3. ^{17}O: Oxygen consumption

Supplying living cells with oxygen is of crucial importance for their viability. This can be seen by the huge impact a shortage of oxygen (hypoxia) has on, for example, brain functions. In order to access the production of NMR visible $H_2{}^{17}O$, the paramagnetic properties of ^{17}O can be used. There are two ways to use ^{17}O in magnetic resonance (MR) experiments.

Firstly, with direct detection of the ^{17}O resonance, and secondly, by use of the change in the ^1H relaxation times due to the coupling between ^{17}O and ^1H. Direct and indirect detections suffer from the low natural abundance of ^{17}O of 0.037%. Together with low values for γ, this leads to a sensitivity which is a factor of 1.7×10^5 lower than for ^1H. To overcome this obstacle, techniques for increasing the ^{17}O concentration are highly valuable. For this purpose, setups, like those listed in reference [23], for the inhalation of ^{17}O enriched gas which can increase the ^{17}O concentration above the natural abundance, are continuously developed.

As mentioned, a concentration increase can be reached by the inhalation of ^{17}O enriched gas. After inhalation, the oxygen binds to haemoglobin due to lung exchange and is transported to the brain via the vascular system. As long as the oxygen gas is bound to haemoglobin, it is practically NMR invisible. In this state, the rotational motion is very slow leading to a very low value for τ_c and therefore to a rapid transverse relaxation. Through cerebral oxygen metabolism ($CMRO_2$), NMR observable ^{17}O enriched water is produced according the following equation:

$$4H^+ + 4e^- + {}^{17}O_2 -> 2H_2{}^{17}O \tag{26}$$

According to references [10] and [24], the relaxation rates R_1 and R_2 for the ^{17}O nucleus in tissue water within the extreme narrowing limit can be estimated as follows:

$$R_2 = \frac{1}{T_2} \cong R_1 = \frac{1}{T_1} = 1.056\chi^2\tau_c \tag{27}$$

where χ is the root mean square coupling constant introduced in Eq. (2). Under coupling to ^{17}O, the transverse relaxation rate $R_{2,H}$ of the ^1H nucleus can be estimated as follows:

$$R_{2,H} = \frac{1}{T_{2,H}} \approx \frac{1}{T_{2,H}^{O}} + \frac{35}{12} P\tau J^2 \tag{28}$$

The relaxation time T_{2H}^{O} denotes the transverse relaxation time for ^{1}H when it is bound to ^{16}O, P is the molar fraction for $H_2{}^{17}O$ which is equivalent to the ^{17}O enrichment factor, τ is in this case the characteristic proton exchange lifetime and J^2 is the scalar ^{17}O-^{1}H coupling constant. Hopkins et al. have shown that only the transverse and not the longitudinal relaxation is influenced by the presence of ^{17}O enriched water [25].

3.4. ^{13}C: Brain metabolites

Like all organic compounds, brain metabolites are consisted of carbon atoms and protons. Therefore, for MRS experiments, it is sensible to consider the carbon isotope ^{13}C, which carries a nuclear spin equal to 1/2. From **Table 1** follows that the value for γ is just 25% of the proton value. Given the low natural abundance of 1.1%, it also has a relatively low NMR sensitivity. If a carbon spectrum is recorded at natural abundance, it will be dominated by the resonances of free fatty acids. Nevertheless, due to the high spectral range of approximately 200 ppm, the spectral resolution of carbon spectra is outstanding. The carbon resonances can be categorized in four groups, which are shown in **Table 6** [4]:

Resonance of nuclei in different CH groups			Resonance of nuclei adjacent to hydroxyl groups	Resonance of nuclei in lipids	Resonance of nuclei in carbonyl groups
$\delta \approx 25 - 60$ ppm			$\delta \approx 60 - 100$ ppm	$\delta \approx 20 - 50$ ppm and $\delta > 120$ ppm	$\delta > 150$ ppm
CH_3 groups	CH_2 groups	CH groups			
$\delta < 25$ ppm	$\delta \approx 25 - 45$ ppm	$\delta \approx 45 - 60$ ppm			

Table 6. Chemical shifts of different ^{13}C moieties.

There are three techniques to increase the sensitivity of the ^{13}C nucleus. One is the application of cryogenic coils where the RF coil is actively cooled by coolant, for example, liquid nitrogen. This reduces the electrical resistance of the coil and increases the signal strength. Another way to increase sensitivity is the application of heteronuclear broadband decoupling. This method also simplifies the interpretation of the spectrum since the scalar coupling between ^{13}C and ^{1}H is lifted. Application of ^{13}C-labelled precursors does not only increase sensitivity. Furthermore, it enables the tracking of brain metabolites, such as glycogen and neurotransmitters [26].

Some examples of detectable metabolites and the chemical shifts of the single carbon atoms are listed in **Table 7** [4]. A very good example for the application of ^{13}C spectroscopy lies in the observation of glycogen regulation. This might have tremendous impact in the understanding of pathologies such as diabetes mellitus. Tracking the metabolic pathways provides a unique information which can only be acquired with the use of ^{13}C spectroscopy.

Metabolite	Atom no.					
	1	2	3	4	5	6
γ-aminobutyric acid (GABA)	182.3	35.2	24.6	40.2	–	–
Glutamate	175.3	55.6	27.8	34.2	182.0	61.4
Glycogen	100.5	–	74.0	78.1	72.1	61.4
N-acetylaspartylglutamic acid (NAA)	179.7	54.0	40.3	179.7	174.3	22.8

Table 7. Chemical shifts (in ppm) of detectable carbon metabolites.

3.5. Functional phantoms and data interpretation

As shown in Section 3.1.4, the main advantage of MQ spectroscopy lies in its capability of recording signals from different coherences simultaneously. However, in order to connect the observed effect to a specific physiological response often remains difficult. In an *in vivo* experiment one has to face the fact that physiological parameters, such as the pH value, temperature, and ion concentrations are hardly, or even not at all accessible. What can be done is, of course, a set of experiments consisting of experiments under pathological conditions and experiments under standard conditions.

A solution to this problem may be found by conducting basic biological experiments, which are carried out on organotypic cell cultures. In contrast to *in vivo* experiments, organotypic cell cultures in microbioreactors provide a high degree of control over the experiment. Specific reactions can be initiated by adding drugs directly to the cell culture.

The principal approach of combining organotypic cell culture experiments in microbioreactors with MRI-detection techniques was impressively shown by Gottwald et al. [3]. In their study, Gottwald et al. used a MRI compatible bioreactor to perform contrast enhanced perfusion ^{1}H-MRI. The setup contained the MRI compatible reactor, which in turn contains a perfused three dimensional cell culture on a chip (3D-KITChip), an external perfusion system with medium supply, and a gas mixing station. It could be shown that the perfusion characteristics are nearly independent of the flow rates, and the system could be completely washed out from applied drugs or contrast agent. From this, it follows that every drug applied in the system will be washed out, allowing the cell culture to reach its initial state again. Basically, this system can serve as a *functional phantom* for the development and testing of new MR sequences, as well as for recording the specific response of cells to different drugs under various physiological conditions.

The bioreactor with a medium reservoir and a peristaltic pump is shown in **Figure 9a**. A cross section of the reactor with the flux of cell culture medium is depicted in **Figure 9b**. One can see that the medium enters the bioreactor housing from below the chip and is then pumped through the pores of the chip, and therefore through the tissue residing in the microcavities, to the compartment above the tissue. The medium finally exits the bioreactor to the right side. By the use of this perfusion technique, the cells can be ideally supplied with medium and can be cultured organotypically for weeks. This setup can then be used to record MQ spectra from the cell culture. An example ^{23}Na-TQTPPI spectrum without cells, recorded with a custom built ^{23}Na surface coil at 9.4 T, is shown in **Figure 9c**. The SQ resonance is shown on the right side of the spectrum. It is not surprising that the SQ resonance is extremely large compared to the rest of the spectrum, since this resonance contains the complete amount of free ions. Higher frequencies are displayed from right to left. It should be noted that despite the DQ suppression, the DQ resonance was not suppressed completely. This is related to imperfection in the excitation pulses arising from the inhomogeneous pulse profile of the surface coil. A zoomed section (shown by the red box) of the spectrum is depicted in **Figure 9d**. As one can see, there is no TQ resonance at the expected frequency.

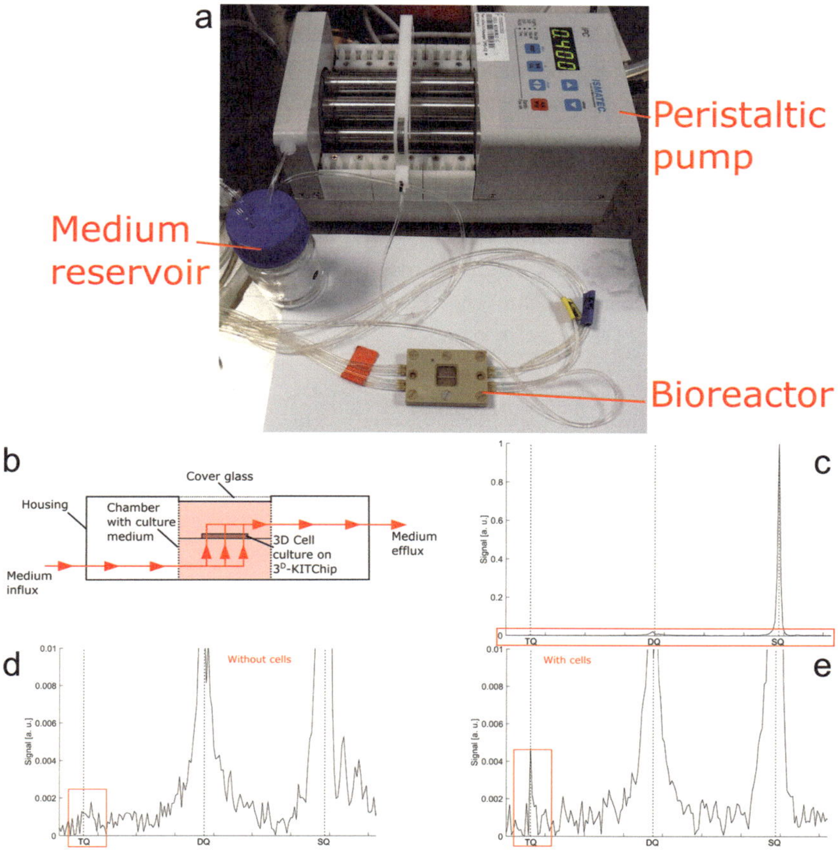

Figure 9. (a) Bioreactor with medium reservoir and peristaltic pump. (b) Cross section of the bioreactor with perfusion direction. (c) With custom built surface coil recorded complete ^{23}Na-TQTPPI spectrum of the bioreactor without cells at 9.4 T. (d) Zoomed section (red box in c) of the spectrum without cells. The spectrum shows no significant TQ contribution. (e) Zoomed section of a ^{23}Na-TQTPPI spectrum with cells. The TQ contribution is clearly present.

The situation changes critically when the experiment is repeated with an active cell culture. In **Figure 9d**, the zoomed section of a ^{23}Na-TQTPPI spectrum is shown from an experiment with a cell culture. One can clearly see the TQ resonance at the expected frequency. Compared to the other resonances, the TQ contribution is extremely small, but the quality of the gained information is revealed if one takes the dimensions of the experiment into account. In the very best case scenario, the entire fraction of the cell culture is approximately 1.2% of the complete volume under investigation. It is obvious that the TQ signal arises from this small fraction which proves that the TQTPPI spectroscopy is a very sensitive tool.

3.6. Conclusions

Based on their involvement in physiological processes such as energy metabolism, generation of action potentials and cell volume regulation, NMR experiments on X-nuclei can provide valuable physiological information.

On the one hand, there are nuclei with a nuclear spin equal to 1/2 which can be measured by means of pulse sequences known from ^{1}H-NMR. For instance, ^{31}P spectra can be generated by usage of simple single pulse sequences. Despite the relative low NMR sensitivity, the information obtained by the application of such simple sequences is always related to the biological background of the nucleus under investigation. On the other hand, for the exploitation of the full potential of spin 3/2 X-nuclei, their unique (quantum) physical properties must be utilised. Sequences capable to generate and record MQCs can be used to study changes in the motional freedom of the nuclei. In living systems, the motional freedom can be influenced by a change in ion binding or by morphological changes of the environment of the nucleus. Therefore, the analysis of MQCs in biological tissue can provide additional information about protein activity or changes in cell volume.

It is of high importance to link changes in the observed signal to the underlying physiological processes. The usage of functional phantoms is a very promising way to establish that link. Since the available magnetic field strength is continuously increasing, the relative low NMR sensitivity of these nuclei may no longer be a drawback in the future.

Author details

Eric Gottwald[1*], Andreas Neubauer[2] and Lothar R. Schad[2]

*Address all correspondence to: eric.gottwald@kit.edu

1 Institute for Biological Interfaces (IBG-5), Karlsruhe Institute of Technology, Karlsruhe, Germany

2 Computer Assisted Clinical Medicine, Medical Faculty Mannheim, Heidelberg University, Mannheim, Germany

References

[1] Konstandin S and Schad LR. 30 Years of Sodium/X-Nuclei Magnetic Resonance Imaging. Magn Reson Mater Phys. 2014;27:1–4.

[2] Konstandin S and Nagel AM. Measurement Techniques for Magnetic Resonance Imaging of Fast Relaxing Nuclei. Magn Reson Mater Phys. 2014;27:5–9.

[3] Gottwald E, Kleintschek T, Giselbrecht S, Truckenmüller R, Altmann B, Worgull M, Döpfert J, Schad LR and Heilmann M. Characterization of a Chip-Based Bioreactor for Three-Dimensional Cell Cultivation via Magnetic Resonance Imaging. Z Med Phys. 2013;23(2):102–110.

[4] de Graaf RA. In Vivo NMR Spectroscopy. 2nd ed. Chichester: John Wiley & Sons Ltd.; 2007. 570 p.

[5] Haacke EM, Brown RW, Thompson MR and Venkatesan R. Magnetic Resonance Imaging. Physical Principles and Sequence Design. John Wiley & Sons Ltd.; 1999. 914 p.

[6] Thulborn KR, Gindin TS, Davis D and Erb P. Comprehensive MR Imaging Protocol for Stroke Management: Tissue Sodium Concentration as a Measure of Tissue Viability in Nonhuman Primate Studies and in Clinical Studies. Radiology. 1999;213(1):156–166.

[7] Umathum R, Rösler MB and Nagel AM. In Vivo ^{39}K MR Imaging of Human Muscle and Brain. Radiology. 2013;269(2):569–576.

[8] Nagel AM, Lehmann-Horn F, Weber MA, Jurkat-Rott K, Wolf MB, Radbruch A, Umathum R and Semmler W. In Vivo ^{35}Cl MR Imaging in Humans: A Feasibility Study. Radiology. 2014;271(2):585–595.

[9] Fuller GF. Nuclear Spins and Moments. J Phys Chem Ref Data 1976;5(4):835–1092.

[10] Abragam A. Principles of Nuclear Magnetism. London: Oxford University Press; 1961. 599 p.

[11] van der Maarel JR. Thermal Relaxation and Coherence Dynamics of Spin 3/2 I. Static and Fluctuating Quadrupolar Interactions in the Multipole Basis. Concept Magn Reson A. 2003;19A(2):97–116.

[12] Dubbers D and Stöckmann H-J. Quantum Physics: The Bottom-Up Approach. From the Simple Two-Level System to Irreducible Representations. 1st ed. Heidelberg, Berlin: Springer-Verlag; 2013. 266 p. DOI: 10.1007/978-3-642-31060-7_1

[13] Rooney WD and Springer Jr CS. A Comprehensive Approach to the Analysis and Interpretations of Resonances of Spins 3/2 from Living Systems. NMR Biomed. 1991;4:209–226.

[14] Schepkin VD, Elumalai M, Kitchen JA, Qian C, Gor'kov PL and Brey WW. In Vivo Chlorine and Sodium MRI of Rat Brain at 21.1 T. Magn Reson Mater Phy. 2014;27(1): 63–70.

[15] Kirsch S, Augath M, Seiffge D, Schilling L and Schad LR. In Vivo Chlorine-35, Sodium-23 and Proton Magnetic Resonance Imaging of the Rat Brain. NMR Biomed. 2010;23:592–600.

[16] Ernst RR, Bodenhausen G and Wokaun A. Principles of Nuclear Magnetic Resonance in One and Two Dimensions. New York, NY: Oxford University Press Inc.; 2004. 610 p.

[17] van der Maarel JR. Relaxation of Spin Quantum Number S = 3/2 Under Multiple-Pulse Quadrupolar Echoes. J Chem Phys. 1991;94(7):4765–4775.

[18] Grant DM and Harris RK, editors. Encyclopedia of Nuclear Magnetic Resonance. 2nd ed. Chichester: John Wiley & Sons Inc.; 1996. 668 p.

[19] Schepkin VD, Odintsov BM, Litvak I, Gor'kov PL, Brey WW, Neubauer A and Budinger TF. Efficient Detection of Bound Potassium and Sodium Using TQTPPI Pulse Sequence. Proc Intl Soc Mag Reson Med. 2015;23:1930.

[20] Meyer RA, Kushmerick TR and Brown R. Application of ^{31}P-NMR Spectroscopy to the Study of Striated Muscle Metabolism. Am J Physiol Cell Ph. 1982;242(1):C1–C11.

[21] Kemp GJ, Meyerspeer M and Moser E. Absolute Quantification of Phosphorus Metabolite Concentration in Human Muscle in Vivo by ^{31}P MRS: A Quantitative Review. NMR Biomed. 2007;20:555–565.

[22] Ng TC, Evanochko WT, Hiramoto RN, Ghanta VK, Lilly MB, Lawson AJ, Corbett, TH, Durant JR and Glickson JD. ^{31}P Spectroscopy of In Vivo Tumors. J Magn Reson. 1982;49:271–286.

[23] Hoffmann SH, Begovatz P, Nagel AM, Umathum R, Schommer K, Bachert P and Bock M. A Measurement Setup for Direct 17O MRI at 7 T. Magn Reson Med. 2001;66:1109–1115.

[24] Zhu XH and Chen W. In Vivo Oxygen-17 NMR for Imaging Brain Oxygen Metabolism at High Field. Prog Nucl Mag Res Sp. 2011;59(4):319–335.

[25] Hopkins AL and Barr RG. Oxygen-17 Compounds as Potential NMR T2 Contrast Agents: Enrichment Effects of H217O on Protein Solutions and Living Systems. Magn Reson Med. 1987;4(4):399–403.

[26] Bachelard H. Landmarks in the Application of ^{13}C-Magnetic Resonance Spectroscopy to Studies of Neuronal/Glial Relationships. Dev Neurosci. 1998;20:277–288.

Chapter 3

Novel Applications of Cardiovascular Magnetic Resonance Imaging-Based Computational Fluid Dynamics Modeling in Pediatric Cardiovascular and Congenital Heart Disease

Margaret M. Samyn and John F. LaDisa

Additional information is available at the end of the chapter

http://dx.doi.org/10.5772/64814

Abstract

Cardiovascular diseases (CVDs) afflict many people across the world; thus, understanding the pathophysiology of CVD and the biomechanical forces which influence CVD progression is important in the development of optimal strategies to care for these patients. Over the last two decades, cardiac magnetic resonance (CMR) imaging has offered increasingly important insights into CVD. Computational fluid dynamics (CFD) modeling, a method of simulating the characteristics of flowing fluids, can be applied to the study of CVD through the collaboration of engineers and clinicians. This chapter aims to explore the current state of the CMR-derived CFD, as this technique pertains to both acquired CVD (i.e., atherosclerosis) and congenital heart disease (CHD).

Keywords: computational, modeling, cardiovascular, atherosclerosis, congenital

1. Introduction

Cardiovascular disease (CVD) is a common cause of morbidity and mortality around the world [1]. Each year, CVD afflicts more than 1.9 million in the European Union and at least 800,000 in the United States of America (USA). The cost of health care has been increasing exponentially over the years with estimates noting about 196 billion Euros per year and 207.3 billion dollars spent annually on direct/indirect costs of cardiovascular disease [1]. In the United States, almost 801,000 Americans died from heart disease, stroke, or other CVD in 2013 and ~85.6 million

Americans live with some form of CVD [1, 2]. While far fewer have congenital heart disease (CHD), these structural problems still afflict about 1% of live-born children and many require intricate operations for treatment/palliation. American Heart Association data suggest that approximately two million Americans live with some form of CHD, as do millions of Europeans and other individuals globally [3].

Mechanical stimuli (such as pressure and strain) have been shown to influence the onset and progression of CVD. For example, wall tension can be estimated as the product of vessel radius and blood pressure (BP). Chronic changes in wall tension initially driven by increases in pressure are believed to be the stimuli for vessel thickening, which then restores wall stress to a preferred operating range [4]. Strain also reflects aortic deformation as present with hypertension and aneurysm formation [5, 6].

Of particular interest is wall shear stress (WSS) (**Figure 1**), which can be generally defined as the frictional force exerted on the walls of a vessel as a result of flowing blood. Areas of low time-averaged WSS are known to correlate with sites of atherogenesis and inflammation from prior studies [7–12]. These studies suggest that specific alterations in mechanical stimuli manifesting from CVD may be the stimuli ultimately leading to morbidity. Hence, there is value in knowing how and when they lead to structural, as well as functional and hemodynamic vascular changes.

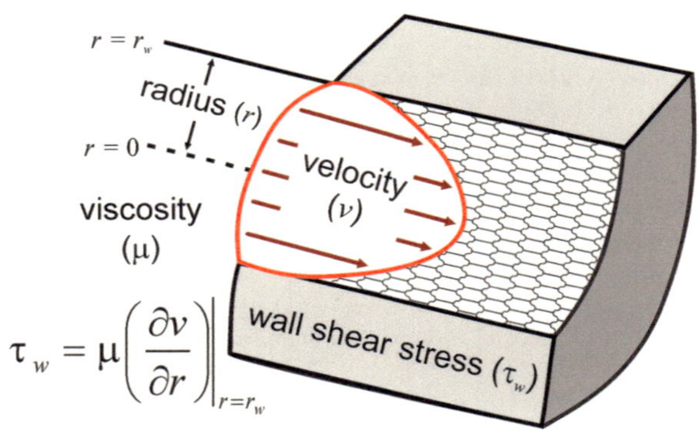

Figure 1. Wall shear stress (WSS). The figure shows schematic illustration of the velocity profile experienced by endothelial cells lining a vessel as a result of flowing blood. WSS (τ_w) can generally be defined as the frictional force exerted on the walls of the vessel. In its simplest form (e.g., plane Couette flow), WSS is the product of viscosity and the near-wall velocity gradient ($\partial v/\partial r$), also known as the shear rate or rate of deformation.

The flow patterns of fluids are governed by partial differential equations that represent conservation laws for quantities such as mass and momentum [13]. Predicting the impact of such flows in biomedical applications, as well as within other scientific disciplines, is time consuming and costly without computational tools. Computational fluid dynamics (CFD) is a method of simulating fluid passing through or around an object, in this case blood vessels, by replacing the partial differential equations with algebraic equations that can be solved numerically using digital computers. There are several open source and commercially available CFD software packages that facilitate the completion of these calculations with user-friendly interfaces that accept various types of medical imaging data. The workflow for each software package then allows a user to generate hemodynamic results (as presented throughout this chapter) with an appreciation for the governing mathematical equations. However, in performing CFD modeling, there are several important clinical and engineering considerations that should be kept in mind.

The general requirements for studying blood flow for patients with CVD and/or CHD using CFD include first creating a model of the vessel geometry from three-dimensional (3D) medical imaging data. Typically, cardiac magnetic resonance (CMR) or computed tomographic (CT) imaging data are readily available 3D data that provide clear definition of anatomy. CFD also requires prescription of the flow information for the entrance and exit of vessels which is gleaned from phase contrast (PC) velocity-encoded CMR data acquired at these sites. It is also necessary to prescribe the hemodynamic state beyond the borders of the 3D imaging dataset in order to obtain physiologic results (e.g., setting downstream resistance to obtain a realistic range of pressure). Direct or indirect assignment of this inlet and outlet information is referred to as "setting the boundary conditions." Rheological properties, such as blood density and viscosity, are then assigned. The last step in the process entails the use of a powerful computer or cluster of computers to solve the governing equations for fluid flow throughout a version of the vessel's geometry, which is represented as a computational mesh.

More specifically, the first step when performing CFD involves creating a computer aided design (CAD) model within the vascular regions of interest from medical imaging data. The CMR imaging focus of the current work most often uses data from either breath-held electrocardiographically (ECG)-gated, magnetic resonance angiography (MRA) or a respiratory-navigated, ECG-gated 3D nongadolinium-enhanced, entire heart CMR sequence. CFD can be used with other sequences and imaging modalities as well. The models created can provide the geometry on a patient-specific basis when it is desirable to focus on a clinical question for a specific patient, or for a group of patients with similar pathology [14]. Alternatively, representative or idealized models are also sometimes used, where the geometry within the idealized model is informed by measurements taken from data within a collection of CMR scans across one or more patients. To date, our workflow has primarily used SimVascular (simvascular.github.io, latest version, La Jolla, CA, USA), but other commonly used software packages that facilitate the import and segmentation of CMR data include Cardiovascular Integrated Modeling and Simulation (CRIMSON, www.crimson.software), the Vascular Modeling Toolkit (VMTK, www.vtnk.org), and Mimics (biomedical.materialise.com/mimics, Plymouth, MI, USA), just to name a few. Each of these programs then facilitates discretization of the CAD model created from CMR data by interacting with some type of meshing software (e.g., MeshSim, www.simmetrix.com, Clifton Park, NY, USA). The parameters selected during the segmentation and meshing steps used in creating a computational version of the vasculature from CMR can have a large impact on the results obtained. For example, the accuracy of WSS indices (see below for details on specific WSS indices of interest) depends greatly on vessel radius, and therefore on the confidence with which segments or 3D boundaries for the CAD model are created from CMR data. In its simplest form (e.g., plane Couette flow), WSS is the product of viscosity and the near-wall velocity gradient (**Figure 1**) [10]. This change in velocity from the wall of an artery to the next nearest location is largely determined by details of the computational mesh that are established. Note that the velocity on the wall is often zero due to a no-slip condition. Unfortunately, the computational costs of obtaining CFD results increase as a function of mesh density. The trade-off is often managed in today's CFD studies by using adaptive-meshing approaches [15, 16] yielding smaller meshes that strategically place more elements where they are most needed, such as near the wall, for improved accuracy when determining WSS.

In practice, the density for blood is typically selected from the literature, and a Newtonian assumption (i.e., constant blood viscosity) is most often employed. Although blood is a shear-thinning fluid, meaning that its viscosity decreases as it is deformed, approximating its behavior as Newtonian is generally thought to be reasonable for the range of shear rates experienced by the portions of the vasculature that are highlighted in the CFD studies below. A unique aspect of CFD software packages designed specifically for biomedical applications is their ability to implement boundary conditions that replicate normal and CVD physiology [17]. For example, the time-varying opposition to blood flow (i.e., impedance spectra) can be calculated from pressure and flow measurements made at the same location in the vascular system, but Windkessel models are often used as an approximation of the impedance given the impracticality of the necessary measurements within a clinical setting [17]. It is an increasingly common CFD modeling standard to employ three-element Windkessel representations derived from CMR-acquired PC velocity-encoded (VENC) flow data for inlet and outlet boundary conditions. More recent boundary condition advancements include cardiac function through the use of closed-loop lumped-parameter networks (LPNs) with CFD models. Closed-loop LPNs were initially developed to model single ventricle physiology [18] and are now being used to characterize flow patterns in the coronary arteries and other vascular regions. These closed-loop LPN models are often tuned to match measured clinical data (i.e., cardiac output (CO), stroke volume, blood pressure, and ejection fraction), and then coupled to patient-specific simulations that use specialized computers to solve the conservation of mass, balance of momentum, and (in some cases) the vessel wall elastodynamics equations [19]. The results are vascular hemodynamic indices that may aid the understanding and care of CVD, following detailed analysis of the resulting indices.

The application of CFD to clinical cardiovascular problems typically requires teamwork between clinicians and engineers, with a step-wise approach to gather and analyze specific data for the study of clinically important blood flow issues (**Figure 2**). As an example, understanding flow in the aortic arch by CFD requires CMR data for the anatomy of interest (MRA or other 3D data), as well as blood flow measurements (from PC velocity-encoded magnetic resonance imaging sequence, PC-MRI) for all major inflow and outflow vessels (in this case, the ascending and descending aortic flow, as well as the brachiocephalic vessels, as denoted by the black dotted lines in **Figure 2**). Blood pressure measurements from each limb are also used in assigning boundary conditions.

When creating CFD models for the aortic arch, the inlet is most often aortic flow. Typically, this can be imposed in one of several representations including plug flow (i.e., uniform flow), parabolic flow (as shown in **Figure 1**), or a patient-specific flow obtained from CMR phase contrast velocity-encoded (PC-MRI) data that intrinsically incorporates elements of both. In vivo, the velocity profile is determined by a ratio of inertial (i.e., those forces driving the flow) to viscous (those forces impeding the flow) forces [17]. If the impact of viscous forces is large, such as in a smaller artery with lower velocity, then the velocity profile will be parabolic. However, in a larger artery such as the aorta, inertial forces are more pronounced, leading to a more uniform velocity profile except near the walls where the impact of viscous forces manifests. It is, therefore, desirable to use a retrospective ECG-gated phase contrast velocity-encoded sequence to sample the velocity profile, which should intrinsically capture these features, downstream of the valve for direct input into a CFD model, but this requires appropriate through-plane and in-plane velocity encoding to adequately resolve flow features. This approach may also be difficult to implement within the typical imaging time available for a clinical case, as it requires specialized sequences and obtains data that are more detailed than that commonly used in clinical imaging. An alternative approach is to construct CFD models with their inlet beginning at the aortic annulus, impose the measured blood flow waveform as an assumed velocity profile at the model inlet (with plug profile or patient-specific flow profile), and allow the curvature and related geometry of the arch to influence the resulting flow patterns [14]. This approach does not require specialized sequences, minimizes the introduction of noise at the model inflow due to inadequate velocity encoding, and allows for improved temporal resolution compared to three-component PC-MRI, using multiple planes for flow assessment [20].

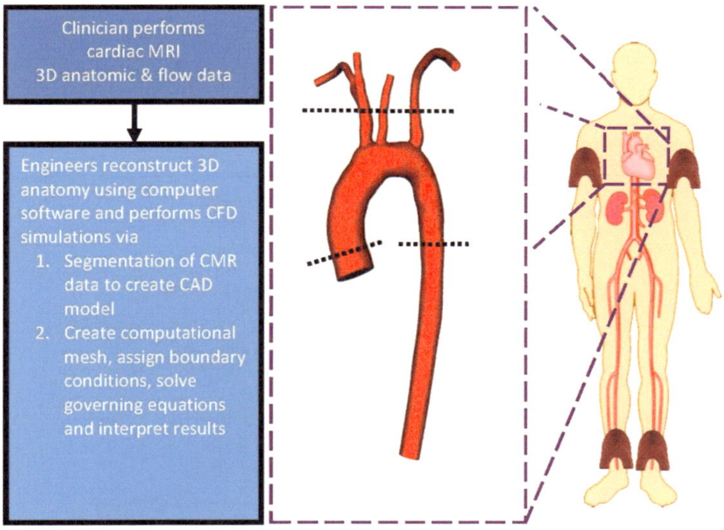

Figure 2. Step-wise creation of computational fluid dynamics (CFD) models. Flow assessments are performed by phase contract magnetic resonance imaging (PC-MRI) at locations noted in the middle panel, while four limb blood pressure assessments are performed after scanning.

In our workflow for CFD simulations of the thoracic aorta to date, which is shown schematically in **Figure 2**, outlet boundary conditions have used measured BP and the PC-MRI flow data from each brachiocephalic vessel and the descending aorta together with an approach called the "pulse pressure method" to assign elements to the Windkessel parameters [21, 22]. The regional resistances, arterial capacitances, and distal resistances are estimated for each case and used in patient-specific modeling (**Table 1**) [23]. Given the very small nature of the intercostal arteries, and the fact that their flow distributions are not typically characterized by imaging, these are not usually employed in the modeling. While flow to the intercostal arteries is important physiologically, characterizing the flow distributions requires multiple phase contrast image acquisition frames or 4D (four-dimensional) blood flow imaging using CMR that is often beyond the time available and needs of the clinically ordered session.

		Control	T1DM
Young's modulus	E (dyn/cm^2)	3.99E+06–3.57E+07	3.23E+06–1.17E+07
Innominate artery	Rc (dyn·s/cm^5)	429–489	320–939
	C (cm^5/dyn)	1.22E–04–1.42E–04	1.23E–04–3.99E–04
	Rd (dyn·s/cm^5)	4250–6500	4520–9260
Left common carotid artery	Rc (dyn·s/cm^5)	687–1720	702–1390
	C (cm^5/dyn)	3.91E–05–1.15E–04	4.94E–05–1.52E–04
	Rd (dyn·s/cm^5)	10,800–19,600	11,800–15,200
Left subclavian artery	Rc (dyn·s/cm^5)	662–1830	500–1480
	C (cm^5/dyn)	6.11E–05–1.26E–04	6.19E–05–1.62E–04
	Rd (dyn·s/cm^5)	6400–23,000	6813–15,000
Descending aortic outlet	Rc (dyn·s/cm^5)	99–231	101–232
	C (cm^5/dyn)	2.67E–04–8.76E–04	2.84E–04–8.16E–04
	Rd (dyn·s/cm^5)	894–4580	1530–4710

With permission and adapted from Samyn et al. [23].

Table 1. Resistances and capacitances used for CFD simulations of adolescent patients [22].

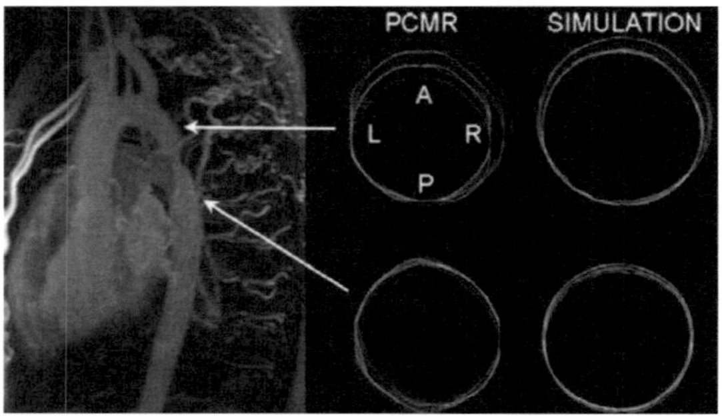

Figure 3. Computational fluid dynamics (CFD) modeling with realistic deformations. A mean intensity projection magnetic resonance angiogram from a patient with aortic coarctation is shown on the left. Temporal wall motion proximal and distal to the coarctation from phase contrast magnetic resonance imaging (PC-MRI) are shown in the middle column, and patient-specific CFD simulations (R = right, L = left, A = anterior, P = posterior) are shown at right.

Fluid-structure interaction (FSI) simulations represent a specialized version of CFD modeling that considers the pulsatility and elastic nature of the arterial system. FSI, therefore, has the potential for introducing more clinically relevant features when determining indices such as instantaneous WSS, time-averaged WSS, and oscillatory shear stress, by including more realistic local deformations (**Figure 3**). For example, considering again the simple case of WSS calculated as the product of the near-wall velocity gradient and viscosity, the movement of the vessel wall as occurs in vivo will impact this calculation. Including local deformations in WSS calculations therefore has the potential to provide more realistic results.

Indices of WSS are calculated from the time-varying velocity field representing flow patterns within the aorta. Blood flow in the aorta, for instance, has long been recognized to be helical and can be replicated by CFD (**Figure 4**) [24]. A helical flow pattern has many positive features including (1) facilitating blood flow transport and suppressing turbulent blood flow, (2) preventing the accumulation of atherogenic low-density lipoprotein (LDL) particles on arterial luminal surfaces, (3) enhancing oxygen transport from the blood to the multilayered arterial wall, (4) reducing the adhesion of platelets and monocytes on the arterial surface, and (5) optimizing flow patterns within origins of the brachiocephalic vessels [25]. Helical blood flow patterns may therefore aid in protecting the arteries from the pathologic mechanisms of atherosclerosis, thrombosis, and intimal hyperplasia, as well as from dilation, aneurysm formation, and dissection [25].

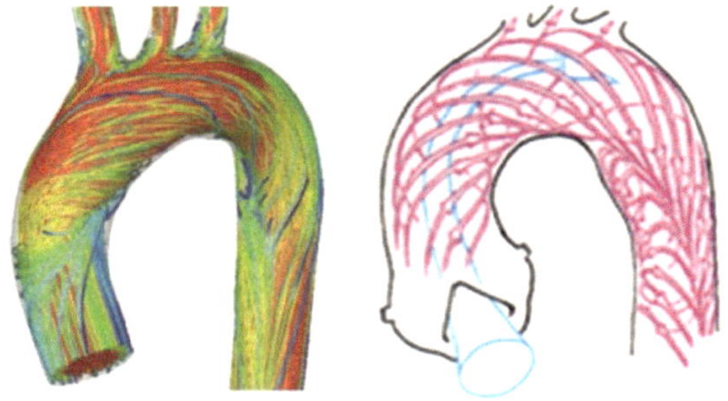

Figure 4. Helical aortic flow. Velocity streamtubes are shown during systole from the simulation of a patient with normal thoracic aortic anatomy (left). The streamtubes replicate the classic patterns elegantly described by Kilner et al. (right) including axially oriented flow during early systole, the development of right-handed helical flow during mid-systole facilitating delivery of blood flow to the arteries of the head and neck, and the presence of complex recirculation regions beginning at end systole [24]. With permission from Wolters-Kluwer journals; Kilner et al. [24].

CFD may offer predictive capabilities for difficult clinical problems as will be discussed in this chapter. For example, MRI during exercise has been pursued since the late 1990s, but is not trivial to implement and is therefore not conducted routinely. More specifically, CMR has been used to quantify blood flow during supine cycle ergometry in the ascending aorta, pulmonary artery [26, 27], abdominal aorta [28, 29], and left ventricle [30]. Indices of WSS and cardiac output were quantified in combination with CFD modeling from a recumbent cycling protocol developed for imaging of the abdominal aorta [31–33]. CFD was also used for patient-specific models of blood flow in the thoracic aorta to quantify indices of WSS under simulated exercise conditions using changes in blood flow and resistance estimated from various literature sources [34, 35]. More recent exercise protocols for use with CMR go one step further. A pilot study developed a protocol to obtain PC-MRI blood flow measurements in the thoracic and brachiocephalic arteries during a three-tiered supine pedaling, and then related these measurements to noninvasive tissue oxygen saturation levels acquired with near-infrared spectroscopy (NIRS) during assessment using the same protocol [36]. The goal of this work was to use NIRS data as a surrogate for exercise PC-MRI data when setting boundary conditions for future CFD studies of the thoracic aorta under simulated exercise conditions. Relationships and ensemble-averaged PC-MRI inflow waveforms are provided in an online repository for this purpose [36].

There are several indices of WSS that have been associated with locations of atherosclerosis in various vascular beds. The most common of these is time-averaged WSS. WSS is actually represented by vectors that change with each fraction of time within the cardiac cycle. Most reports simply present time-average representations on the wall within the region of interest; this is done for simplicity and because the mechanisms and details by which a particular WSS index leads to neo-intimal thickening are not yet precisely known. Areas of low time-averaged WSS have also been found in a rotating pattern down the descending aorta [37], correlate with areas of plaque deposition [38], and are accentuated after correction of CoA [14]. However, there is evidence suggesting that temporal and spatial changes in WSS may also serve as stimuli for neo-intimal thickening. Oscillatory shear index (OSI) is also commonly reported in CFD studies [11]. OSI is a measure of WSS directionality in which lower OSI values indicate that WSS is oriented predominantly in the primary direction of blood flow, while a value of 0.5 is indicative of bidirectional WSS with a time-average value of zero. Theoretically, regions of low WSS magnitude and high OSI are less likely to experience fluid forces that promote washout of noxious and potentially atherogenic materials in contact with the arterial surface (e.g., LDL). In general, adverse values for these WSS indices (e.g., ~15 dyn/cm^2 for the thoracic aorta) are expressed as thresholds for low magnitude instantaneous and time-averaged WSS. OSI greater than 0.1 are considered adverse, as are spatial and temporal WSS gradients greater than 100 dyn/cm^2 and ±200 dyne/cm^2/s, respectively) [12, 21, 39, 40]. Understanding these hemodynamic principles and differences between indices that use them, the practitioner may apply CFD modeling to describe blood flow patterns in the setting of typical clinical cardiovascular pathology—atherosclerosis and congenital heart disease.

Any discussion of CFD for use in generating flow patterns and indices of WSS would be remiss without a discussion of potential limitations, particularly with respect to advancements in CMR that have facilitated quantification of the same indices through direct processing of data from a more advanced clinical imaging session. For example, 4D blood flow imaging using CMR has been used to investigate flow disruptions in the thoracic aorta [37, 41, 42]. These methods do require specialized pulse sequences that may be outside of the clinical workflow for some centers, are complex to acquire and post-process, and prolong scan time (~15–20 min for a 4D-navigated flow-imaging dataset). Additionally, these methods suffer from low spatial/temporal resolution relative to CFD simulations, which could limit the precision of the WSS results compared to those WSS data calculated from a properly conducted CFD simulation where uncertainties in the processes employed were appropriately considered [43–45]. For example, the limitations and variability in the model creation process must be carefully controlled by acquiring a high-resolution 3D representation of the anatomy (by MRA or equivalent sequence) and PC-MRI data. Furthermore, the individuals building CAD models must be rigorous when using software, especially with regard to selection of a mesh of sufficiently high density. In this manner, there can generally be a high level of confidence in the results assuming that physiologic boundary conditions have been implemented. WSS results from 4D blood flow imaging can suffer from the same potential limitations of traditional CFD modeling techniques, if the spatial resolution and post-processing operations do not carefully capture the near-wall velocity gradient.

Additional limitations may exist when CFD modeling is attempted for biologic systems. First, clinical acquisition of suboptimal 3D anatomic data can adversely affect models. Acquisition of non-robust 3D data may lead to oversimplification of anatomy during modeling. Second, suboptimally acquired PC-MRI flow data, with inadequate temporal resolution or low dynamic range, may underestimate flow. Third, ignoring cardiac motion, which can affect the accuracy of flow determinations, may lead to errors in modeling [46]. Finally, assigning accurate boundary conditions (especially resistances of the peripheral vasculature or the microcirculation when coronary modeling is attempted) can be challenging, as detailed information may have to be gleaned from the literature because patient-specific data may be difficult to attain. Such resistances can also vary over time and certainly may differ in healthy and diseased states [47].

2. Computational fluid dynamics modeling applied to the study of atherosclerosis

Atherosclerosis is a complex pathobiologic process which begins with endothelial dysfunction, involves a cascade of particles (including white blood cells, chemotactic factors, and smooth muscle cells), and leads to progressive changes in blood vessel walls (**Figure 5**) [48].

After the initial endothelial dysfunction, atherosclerotic plaque develops over many years [49, 50]. The initial feature in the evolution of plaque, seen on autopsy in children as young as 10–18 years old, is the fatty streak [51]. Many studies have shown that intimal thickening, as assessed by ultrasound, can be detected as plaque burden increases. At first, plaque causes outward remodeling of a blood vessel, maintaining the lumen's dimensions, followed by plaque encroachment on the vessel lumen [52]. By the time atherosclerotic plaque causes stenosis (and decreases luminal dimensions by 60% or more), symptoms can be seen under conditions of great oxygen demand, such as exercise. Thus, if the carotid vasculature is affected, cerebral transient ischemic attacks might be manifested, whereas if the coronaries are affected, then myocardial ischemia can occur and be manifested as angina. Peripheral plaque can lead to symptoms of left pain—either claudication or rest pain.

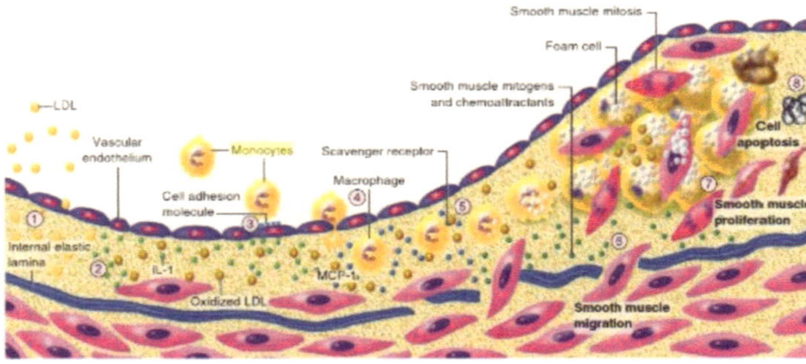

Figure 5. Atherosclerosis. Schematic representation of the evolution of the atherosclerotic plaque. (1) Accumulation of lipoprotein particles in the intima. The modification of these lipoproteins is depicted by the darker color. Modifications include oxidation and glycation. (2) Oxidative stress, including products found in modified lipoproteins, can induce local cytokine elaboration (green spheres). (3) The cytokines thus induced increase the expression of adhesion molecules (blue stalks on endothelial surface) for leukocytes that cause their attachment and chemoattractant molecules that direct their migration into the intima. (4) Blood monocytes, on entering the artery wall in response to chemoattractant cytokines, such as monocyte chemoattractant protein 1 (MCP-1), encounter stimuli such as macrophage colony-stimulating factor (M-CSF) that can augment their expression of scavenger receptors. (5) Scavenger receptors mediate the uptake of modified lipoprotein particles and promote the development of foam cells. Macrophage foam cells are a source of mediators, such as further cytokines and effector molecules such as hypochlorous acid, superoxide anion (O_2^-), and matrix metalloproteinases. (6) Smooth muscle cells (SMCs) migrate into the intima from the media. (7) SMCs can then divide and elaborate extracellular matrix, promoting extracellular matrix accumulation in the growing atherosclerotic plaque. In this manner, the fatty streak can evolve into a fibrofatty lesion. (8) In later stages, calcification can occur (not depicted) and fibrosis continues, sometimes accompanied by SMC death (including programmed cell death, or apoptosis) yielding a relatively acellular fibrous capsule surrounding a lipid-rich core that may also contain dying or dead cells and their detritus (IL-1 = interleukin-1; LDL = low-density lipoprotein) [48]. With permission from Elsevier Health Science.

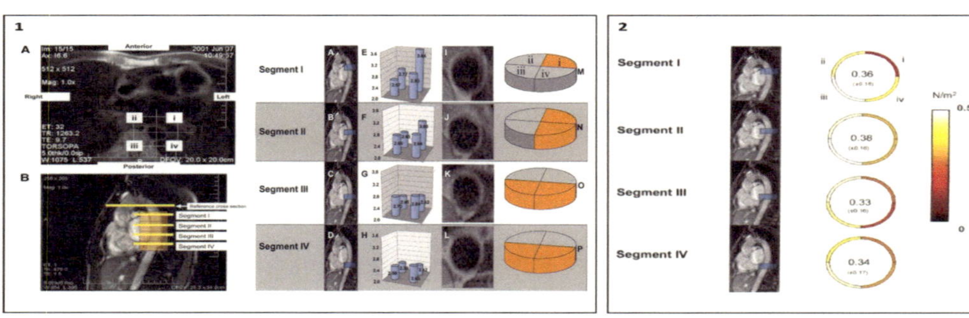

Figure 6. Shear stress and plaque distributions depend on axial and circumferential location. In the upper corner of panel 1, Image A shows circumferential designation (i–iv), while the lower left image (Image B) shows each axial location of the aorta studied. Plaque distribution is shown as pie charts for each segment. On the right (panel 2), shear stress is shown [38]. With permission from Wentzel et al. [38].

Studies have emerged to characterize the vascular hemodynamic effects of plaque by employing computational modeling based on CMR data. This area of CFD research attempts to systematically study vascular WSS and OSI as a way to better understand where plaque forms and how plaque influences blood flow. In a study of adults with preexisting aortic plaque, for example, time-averaged WSS patterns existed in a rotating pattern down the thoracic aorta that correlated with areas of atherosclerotic plaque [38]. WSS distribution, therefore, depended on the axial level and circumferential location in a given axial level of the aorta (**Figure 6**). Similarly, many other CFD studies have shown low WSS and high OSI are associated with atherosclerosis. In an adult coronary CT study, coronary segments with established plaque exhibited lower WSS compared to adjacent normal areas [53]. Within plaques, WSS was lower, and plaque volume was higher in mid-plaque compared to upstream and downstream areas (**Figure 7**) [53]. In a study of carotid atherosclerosis, low time-averaged WSS and high OSI were seen in areas of increased mature plaque volume (**Figure 8**) [54].

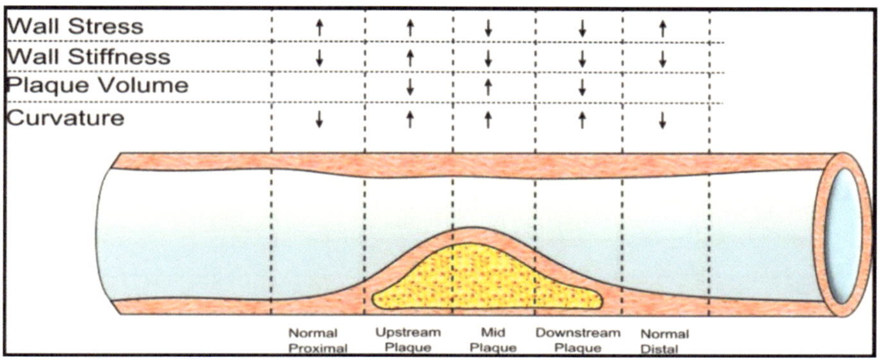

Figure 7. Variation of wall stress (WS), wall stiffness, plaque volume, and curvature along a plaque (note that within plaques, wall shear stress was lower and plaque volume higher in mid-plaque compared to upstream and downstream areas) [53]. With permission from Katranas et al. [53].

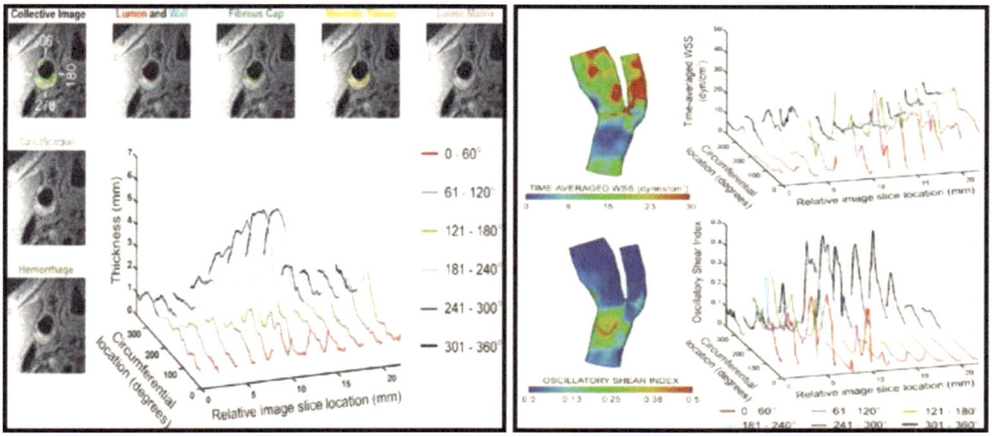

Figure 8. Carotid plaque and wall shear stress. In areas of mature plaque (left), low time-average wall shear stress (right, top right) and high oscillatory sheer index (right, bottom right) are seen [54]. With permission and adapted from LaDisa et al. [54].

This prior work served as motivation for a novel pilot CMR study of early vascular changes in pediatric patients with type 1 diabetes. Twenty preadolescent and adolescent patients with type 1 diabetes (median age of 15.8 years, range of 11.6–18.4 years) were enrolled in this prospective CMR study and compared with eight control subjects (15.8 years with a range of 10.3–18.2 years). Using same-day brachial artery reactivity testing, lower flow-mediated dilation was seen for the subjects with diabetes ($p = 0.036$), as expected—indicating the presence of endothelial dysfunction in this group, as seen by others [55]. When patient-specific CFD models were created from CMR data, those with diabetes had more aortic regions with high time-averaged WSS when compared with controls, although the groups had similar OSI (**Figure 9**) [23]. Many cardiovascular risk factors, including type 1 diabetes, induce physiological outward arterial remodeling (dilation) that begins in response to overall higher initial laminar shear stress (Glagov phenomenon). With vascular inflammation, remodeling progresses, resulting in adverse shear stress in larger arteries [56]. This pilot pediatric diabetes study may provide a glimpse into early vascular remodeling (i.e., where wall shear stress is still high and the aorta, which has begun to stiffen, has yet to dilate). Longitudinal studies are needed to understand how areas of WSS and OSI change with aging, and as atherosclerosis progresses. Understanding this may enhance therapies for early treatment of atherosclerosis by aiding the development of medications that favorably alter WSS and OSI [23].

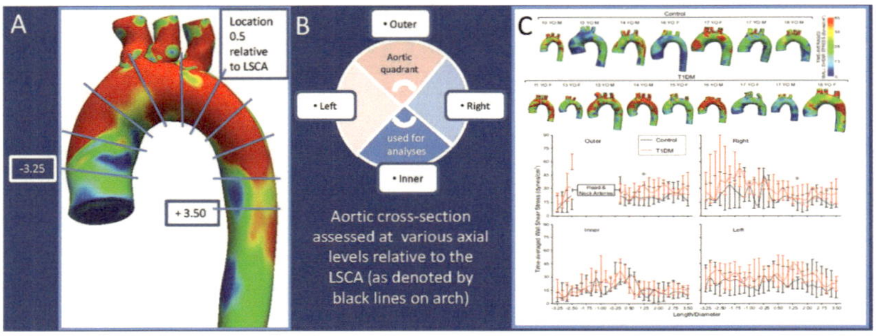

Figure 9. Regional differences in time-average wall shear stress for children with type 1 diabetes (red line) versus controls (black line) are shown (graphs in panel C). Panel A shows the time-averaged wall shear stress (TAWSS) display for a representative patient with type 1 diabetes (T1DM) with blue lines showing where assessments were made relative to the left subclavian artery (LSCA). Panel B shows the circumferential locations assessed. These are displayed graphically in panel C. Along right, left, outer, and, to a lesser degree, the inner curvatures of the aorta, the median time-averaged wall shear stress (TAWSS) at each location for diabetics (red line on the graphs) tended to be higher than median TAWSS for controls (black line), reaching significance at two locations, one along the outer curvature (location 1.25) and another along the anatomic right side (location 1.5) of the aorta [23]. With permission and adapted from Samyn et al. [23].

3. Computational fluid dynamics modeling and congenital heart disease

CFD modeling is useful in understanding not only blood flow as it relates to atherosclerosis but also blood flow in a number of structural heart diseases, including aortic coarctation (CoA), aortic dilation, and aneurysms (as with bicuspid aortic valve and connective tissues diseases), and for more complex diseases, such as repaired Tetralogy of Fallot (TOF) (to aid percutaneous interventions) and single ventricle physiology (to optimize the Fontan operation's total cavopulmonary palliation). Collaboration between clinicians and engineers is important, so that optimal workflow can be achieved to allow timely, patient-specific model creation for consideration in clinical decision making. **Table 2** shows some situations where CFD simulations have been applied to clinical cardiovascular medicine; these will be discussed here.

Area of interest	Applications	Clinical impact	Limitations
Coronary artery disease (CAD)	Models based on angiography or CT scan may predict hemodynamically important plaque.	Models allow virtual stenting to optimize treatment.	Accurate coronary vessel reconstructions and patient-specific boundary conditions (myocardial resistance) are challenging to simulate.
Aorta Aneurysm Dissection Coarctation	Models quantify hemodynamics to develop optimal therapy and predict outcome.	Models may be used to predict aneurysm progression and risk of rupture and may aid in patient follow-up by reducing additional imaging. Models may aid care by allowing appropriate planning and may contribute to stent design.	Wall motion and low image contrast between vessel wall and thrombus may affect modeling, but fluid structure interaction (FSI) may aid analyses.
Arterial wall	Models determine local wall shear stress (WSS) and oscillatory shear index (OSI) related to atherosclerosis.	Models may predict plaque, note sites likely of rupture, and allow optimization of therapy with medications/ devices (i.e., stents).	Detailed anatomy of some circulations may be challenging to model; using accurate boundary conditions can be challenging.
Congenial Heart Diseases Coarctation Single ventricle Tetralogy of Fallot	Models aid understanding of blood flow in complex heterogeneous diseases and may aid therapy.	Modeling will allow prediction of hemodynamic response to possible surgical- and device-based treatments which sometimes dramatically alter the circulation.	Some have cited this as the "ultimate personalization challenge" given the heterogeneous nature of each category of CHD, the complex anatomy, and patient-specific boundary conditions needed.

With permission and adapted from Morris et al. [47].

Table 2. Applications of CFD modeling to cardiac disease [46].

3.1. Aortic CFD modeling for congenital heart diseases

Building upon the CFD modeling efforts summarized above that focused on the thoracic aorta as a vascular surrogate for the coronaries in the study of atherosclerosis, CFD modeling research naturally extended to the diseases of the thoracic aorta—especially to the study of CoA. CoA is a relatively common congenital narrowing of the proximal thoracic aorta, occurring in about 8–11% of patients with CHD, and usually involves the thoracic aorta just after the origin of the left subclavian artery (juxta-ductal CoA). Patients with unrepaired CoA may suffer from ill-effects of hypertension (or in infancy, from cardiovascular collapse with ductal closure). Even after successful CoA repair, many are followed due to the presence of bicuspid aortic valve (up to 85%) with or without stenosis, residual hypertension (7–33% of patients) [57], re-coarctation (5–50%) [58], aortic aneurysm, aortic dissection, and possibly early atherosclerosis [59]. Recent CFD modeling studies have shown altered time-average WSS after end-to-end anastomoses [14]. CFD modeling has also been employed to assess WSS after Dacron patch repair of CoA [60]—an operative procedure now known to be complicated by aneurysm formation. Aneurysms, in turn, introduce local geometric abnormalities leading to heterogeneity in WSS that have historically been linked to adverse consequences such as cellular proliferation and plaque progression (**Figure 10**). Bicuspid aortic valve is a frequently found coexisting CHD for patients with CoA—occurring in up to 85% of these individuals. Recently, sophisticated CFD simulations, using a custom MATLAB® program (MathWorks, Natick, MA, USA) to facilitate segmentation of a common variant (right-left cusp fusion) of bicuspid aortic valve, attempted to account for the influence of the valve on flow patterns and turbulence in the ascending aorta [61]. This represents an added step toward realism, and constitutes an alternative to imposing measured PC-MRI data directly when creating patient-specific CFD models for patients with CoA and bicuspid aortic valve. Additionally, attempts to account for cardiac motion have been applied to the study of aortic flow patterns via CFD. Cardiac motion seems to be most prevalent in altering ascending aortic (AAo) flow rather than flow in the arch or descending aortic flow, likely due in part to less tissue tethering for AAo than the descending aorta [46]. Differences in time-averaged WSS quantified in this study from simulations with the measured PC-MRI inflow waveforms, as compared to motion-compensated cardiac waveforms, were more pronounced than differences from the model creation or mesh dependent aspects of CFD discussed above. These results suggest that accounting for cardiac motion when quantifying blood flow through the aortic valve can lead to different conclusions for hemodynamic indices, which may be important, if these results are ultimately used to predict patient outcomes [46]. CFD modeling may, thus, aid in optimal management of aortic and aortic arch diseases—whether by influencing operative technique or optimizing devices through material development.

Modeling can aid analysis of aortic dilation, which occurs in patients with bicuspid aortic valves, or in those with connective tissue diseases, such as Marfan, Loeys-Dietz, and Ehlers Danlos syndromes. It is unclear if this is causal, or, more likely, contributing to the underlying vascular pathology. In these populations, CFD has demonstrated adversely high OSI in the ascending aorta, an area prone to dilation [62]. Many of these patients undergo an operation to treat an excessively dilated aorta, in order to prevent aortic rupture. Operative techniques used might include total aortic root and valve replacement (TAR), valve-sparing root replacement (VSRR), or the novel and less invasive procedure of placing a personalized external aortic root support (PEARS) introduced by Golesworthy et al. [63]. Using MRI-derived data for CFD modeling, Marfan patients have recently been studied after operation for placement of PEARS, and although qualitative hemodynamic indices appeared similar, some small differences in quantitative measures of helical flow were seen pre- and post PEARS in a small cohort. Larger, longitudinal studies will be needed to understand the hemodynamic effects of these operations. CFD may be used in the future to optimize therapy [64] by aiding the creation of aortic "sleeves" from materials which impart better WSS properties to the patients.

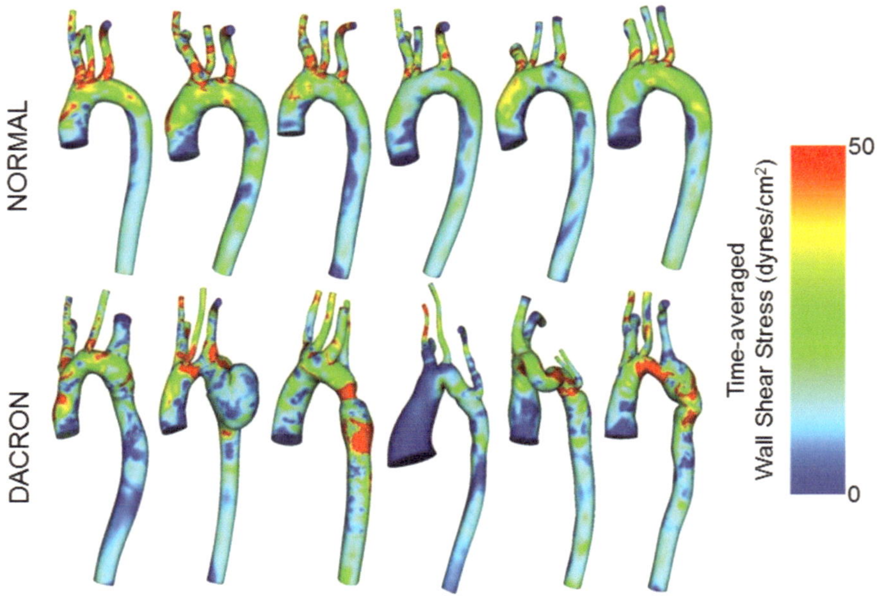

Figure 10. CFD for arch repair by Dacron patch. Time-averaged WSS distributions in six normal subjects (top, 5M, 1F ages 25–33 years) as well as age- and gender-matched patients previously treated for CoA by Dacron patch aortoplasty (below).

3.2. Single ventricle CFD modeling

Over the last decade, CFD modeling has increasingly been applied to patients with single ventricle physiology (**Table 3**), who often require multiple palliative operations in infancy and childhood. The goal of operative therapy is to have the functioning ventricle as the systemic pump, and to secure a source of pulmonary blood flow. Unobstructed flow to the systemic and pulmonary circulations is the goal—to achieve widely patent branch pulmonary arteries and no residual aortic arch obstruction [65].

When the aorta is small, as in hypoplastic left heart syndrome (HLHS), shortly after birth, the infant is palliated with a Norwood operation to create a neo-aorta from side-side anastomosis of the main pulmonary artery (MPA) and native aorta. Usually, arch repair is undertaken in the same setting. Atrial septectomy occurs too - to allow mixing of systemic and pulmonary venous flow, and pulmonary flow is guaranteed by either an aortopulmonary arterial shunt (i.e., either a Blalock-Taussig (BT) or a central shunt) or right ventricular (RV) to pulmonary shunt (i.e., the Sano shunt). Some time between 3 and 6 months' of age, when the pulmonary vascular resistance is acceptable, the patient undergoes cavo-pulmonary shunt (**Figure 11**) to direct a portion of the systemic venous blood to the lungs for oxygenation. Finally, when the child is older (18 months to 4 years of age), the remaining systemic venous blood and hepatic blood are directed to the lungs via completion of the Fontan (**Figure 12**). CMR is often used in clinical follow-up of these patients.

RV morphology	LV morphology	RV or LV morphology
• Hypoplastic left heart syndrome (HLHS) • Complex double outlet RV	• Tricuspid atresia • Pulmonary atresia • Doublet inlet LV • Severe Epstein's anomaly	• Unbalanced AV canal defect • Straddling or criss-cross AV valve connections • Heterotaxy

With permission from Johnson et al. [65].

Table 3. Single ventricular anatomy [65].

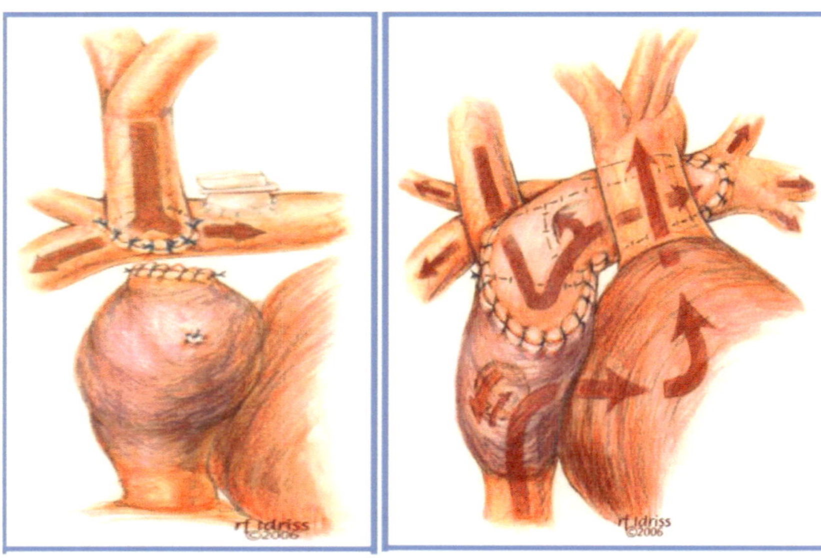

Figure 11. Cavo-pulmonary shunts of the Glenn circuit (left, current era) and Hemi-Fontan (right, original operative technique [66]. With permission from Pelletier et al. CTSNet.org. 2013.

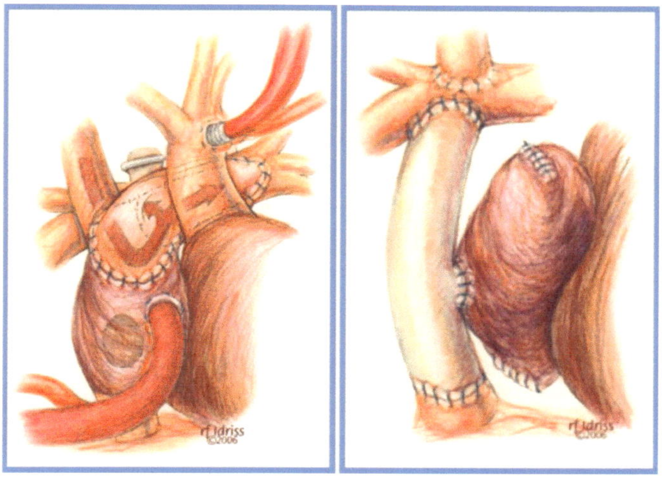

Figure 12. Fontan circulations—various adaptations. "Classic Fontan" (left) has a "classic Glenn circuit" plus an anastomosis of the right atrial appendage to the left pulmonary artery (LPA). Lateral tunnel Fontan (not shown) uses a baffle within the right atrium to partition systemic and pulmonary venous blood, allowing for child's growth. Extracardiac conduit Fontan (right) uses a tube graft to connect IVC to Glenn (SVC/PA), and is often fenestrated [67]. With permission from Jacobs et al. CTSNet.org. 2013.

Using CMR data, CFD modeling in single ventricle patients has focused on understanding energy losses occurring in these unique low-velocity flow Glenn and Fontan circuits. Modeling has aimed to understand blood flow distribution to the lungs by using branch pulmonary arterial PC-MRI data in CFD models. In this manner, CFD has also led to a better understanding of the pulmonary distribution of hepatic flow and the elusive "hepatic factor" which has been implicated in the development of pulmonary arteriovenous malformations [68–72].

Catheterization-based CFD modeling, such as that included in the work by Migliavacca et al. [73], has advanced the clinicians' understanding of the unique Norwood circulation by showing that (1) larger shunts diverted an increased proportion of cardiac output to the lungs and away from systemic perfusion, resulting in poorer oxygen delivery and pulmonary overcirculation, and that (2) the systemic vascular resistance exerted more effects on hemodynamics than pulmonary vascular resistance. CMR-based CFD modeling efforts have been less common in this Norwood population, because of a number of challenges. First, highly turbulent flow from shunts (BT, central or Sano) can lead to inaccuracies in modeling, because of suboptimal PC-MRI data. Second, as this Norwood population is very young ages (i.e., neonates to a few months of age), often 3D anatomic imaging data (CMR or CT) are not readily available, as it is not typically acquired during routine clinical care, which relies predominantly on echocardiographic data. Finally, without catheterization data simultaneous with 3D anatomic imaging, accurate pulmonary and systemic resistance data may not be available, thereby leading to inaccuracies in CFD modeling. Furthermore, the influences of anesthesia (used during catheterization or 3D image acquisition) on such resistance data may lead to models that may not adequately represent real-life clinical conditions. Nonetheless, computational modeling of this unique Norwood physiology has been attempted and refined over the last two decades [74] with a nice review of the challenges provided by Pennati et al. [75].

CFD modeling of cavo-pulmonary shunts has been more limited relative to the CFD study of the total cavo-pulmonary shunt (Fontan). In pilot research, the Stanford Institute for Computational and Mathematical Engineering, though, systematically studied five Glenn patients, incorporating CMR data and catheterization data into their CFD models. Inflow data came from the superior vena cava (SVC) PC-MRI flow data, while outflow data were more complex and depended on the patient's specific pulmonary tree. They first determined right and left lung flow split from the right pulmonary artery (RPA) and the left pulmonary artery (LPA) PC-MRI flow data and then determined the total resistance—i.e., R_p (proximal resistance) plus R_d (distal resistance) for the pulmonary tree. They calculated the mean flow in each branch as being proportional to the outlet surface area and calculated the downstream resistance by the mean pressure gradient (obtained at catheterization) between SVC and left atrium. The authors show low WSS, complex Glenn flow patterns at the caval-pulmonary anastomoses with a transition to laminar flow more distally in the lung, and a complex pressure waveform which dampens after the anastomoses. Power loss in this small cohort was low, and the efficiency of flow was high. The complexity of the pulmonary tree seems to add computational time, but more work is needed to understand how many pulmonary branches should be modeled for accuracy. This study highlights the complexity of assigning appropriate inlet and outlet boundary conditions—a problem that is compounded when patients are studied by either CMR or cardiac catheterization while they are under anesthesia which alters systemic and pulmonary resistances [76].

CFD may be useful for bilateral bidirectional Glenn connections [77], where patients have the persistence of the left and right superior vena cava. Case reports of CFD modeling in this unique Glenn circuit show differential lung flow due to differences in pulmonary resistance (which may result, e.g., from unilateral lung disease (e.g., pneumonia)) or differences in branch pulmonary arterial dimensions. Furthermore, de Zelicourt et al. [78] have noted that unbalanced lung perfusion may affect pulmonary arterial growth. Thus, constructing the best Glenn circuit with attention to downstream branch pulmonary arterial flow may be essential to long-term patient health.

Surgeons have always tried to avoid "right angles" in the construct of the unique bidirectional Glenn and Fontan circuits, as they perceived unfavorable flow disturbances in these regions. de Leval et al. [79, 80] described various methods for palliation of HLHS. In 2007, Bove et al. [81] studied Fontan circuits of different varieties using computational simulations and showed that when either the total cavo-pulmonary connection (TCPC) or the extra cardiac connection (ECC) is performed after a bidirectional Glenn anastomosis, caval offset of the superior and inferior vena cavae (IVC) can be achieved by beveling the IVC portion of the connection to either the right or the left lung. They demonstrated that beveling the TCPC to the right conferred a significant advantage to the TCPC. Similarly, when the ECC was beveled toward the left lung, important differences were found in flow distribution, but not power losses. This research has been continued by many with continued scrutiny regarding possible power losses in this low-velocity circuit, which is prone to swirling of blood flow due to competitive flow from the superior and inferior vena cavae [81, 82]. Some centers, such as the Children's Hospital of Philadelphia and Stanford University, among others, have conducted "virtual operative procedures" to study the hemodynamic effects of a given operation by employing CMR-based CFD modeling techniques. These computations have led some to alter the Fontan circuit by employing a "Y graft" for the Fontan [83], as first described by two groups—Marsden et al. [84] and Soerensen et al. [85]. Not only is the energy loss reduced, especially during simulated exercise, but also IVC flow (and the seemingly critical "hepatic flow") can be more equally distributed to the right and left lung fields, which is potentially protective against the development of pulmonary arteriovenous malformations (**Figure 13**) [83, 85, 86].

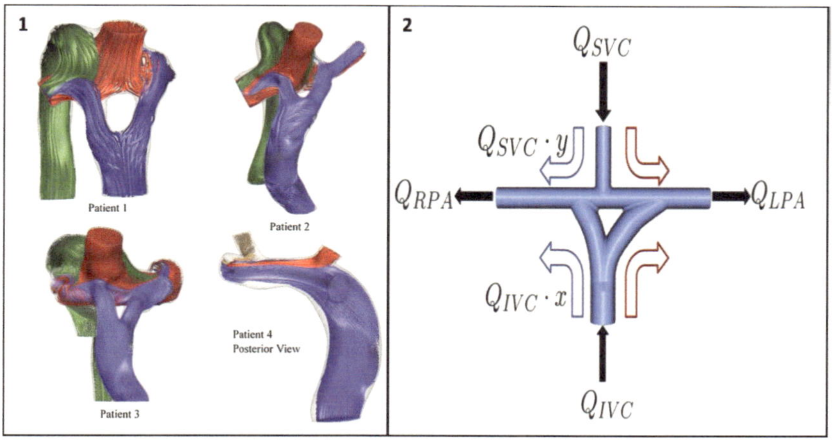

Figure 13. A novel variation in Fontan circuit [83, 86]. Panel 1 shows color representations of the blood flow from azygous vein (green), Glenn circuit (red), and inferior vena cava into the two arms of the Fontan Y graft (blue). Panel 2 gives blood flow calculations for this "Y graft", based on conservation of mass; thus, QRPA = QIVC • x + QSVC • y and QLPA = QIVC • $(1 - x)$ + QSVC • $(1 - y)$, where x is the fraction of hepatic flow going to the RPA and y is the fraction of SVC flow going to the RPA (SVC, superior vena cava; IVC, inferior vena cava; RPA, right pulmonary artery; LPA, left pulmonary artery; Q, flow rate). With permission and adapted from Haggerty et al. [83] and Yang et al. [86].

3.3. Tetralogy of Fallot CFD modeling

Patients with Tetralogy of Fallot (TOF) (i.e., subpulmonary and/or pulmonary valve stenosis with ventricular septal defect, overriding aorta, and right ventricular (RV) hypertrophy) typically undergo operative repair in infancy. Long term, their outcome is related to the degree of chronic pulmonary regurgitation (PR) (i.e., pulmonary valve leakage), and resulting RV dilation and RV dysfunction. Restrictive RV physiology correlates with larger RV and more PR after repair [87]. Pulmonary arterial compliance impacts the amount of regurgitation [88]. Thus, establishing and maintaining appropriate sized branch pulmonary arteries is essential, as elevated resistance distal to compliant arteries exacerbates PR. Furthermore, the initial type of TOF repair may impact how much PR a patient has—with those having RV outflow tract (RVOT) transannular patches having considerably more PR and more dilated RV than those with RV—pulmonary arterial conduits [89]. Patients with repaired TOF, in the current era, are frequently studied by CMR to better understand when the PR has progressed sufficiently to warrant operative intervention for pulmonary valve replacement [90].

CMR-based CFD modeling has been applied to the study of TOF patients to understand how branch pulmonary arterial geometry (i.e., diameters and the bifurcation angles for the right and left pulmonary arteries) influences pulmonary regurgitation (**Figure 14**) [91, 92]. Chern et al. found that regurgitation occurs first from the LPA and suggested that it may be due to the small angle between LPA and MPA. The authors acknowledge the limitations of their CFD models which do not account for the influences of either distal pulmonary vascular resistance or ventricular hypertrophy (diastolic pressure) on pulmonary regurgitation.

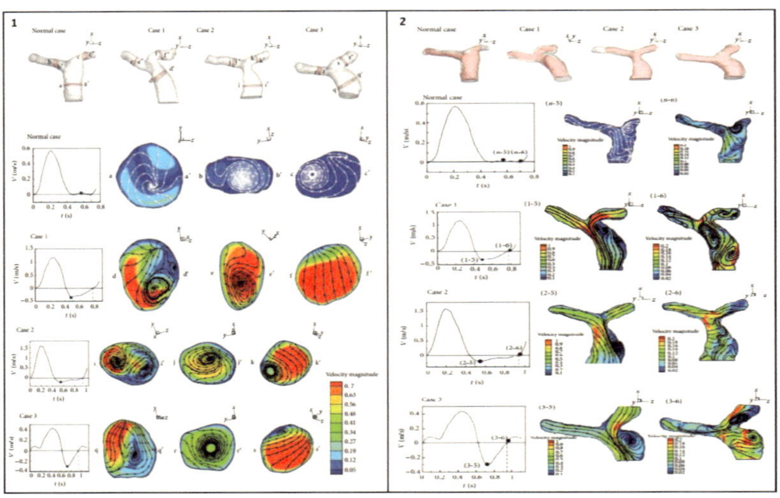

Figure 14. Numerical study of blood flow in pulmonary arteries after repair of Tetralogy of Fallot with different flow patterns in diastole based on angle of bifurcation. 1. Cross-sectional flow patterns and velocity distributions are shown for minimum velocity in the cardiac cycle (as noted by the black dot on the graph). 2. Flow patterns and velocity distributions shown at the minimum flow location and at end diastole (as noted by the black dots on the graph) [93]. With permission and adapted from Chern et al. [93].

Some researchers have proposed that a "reference geometry atlas" be available for the branch pulmonary arteries onto which specific patient data (derived from CMR 3D MRA imaging) may be mapped, so as to reduce computational time [92]. This is a novel idea that may allow CFD to move more readily from the research realm to clinical setting. Others have described in silico models to permit "virtual surgery" for patients with TOF and left pulmonary arterial stenosis [94], an intriguing application that warrants further CFD study with larger cohorts. Another novel application of CFD for patients with repaired TOF is modeling of the RVOT flow to target those for whom transcatheter pulmonary valve replacement is not currently the ideal intervention due to RVOT dilation. In this manner, CFD may aid the design of novel percutaneously placed "pulmonary valve reducer" (for those with enlarged RVOT) [95], thus allowing nonoperative pulmonary valve replacement. Additional CFD research for TOF patients is warranted as better solutions are sought for this population that has chronic PR.

4. Conclusions

In summary, creating clinically relevant CFD models requires care and rigor by individuals at all steps in the process—from initial acquisition of clinical data through all the steps of mathematical modeling. CFD is moving beyond being simply an intriguing mathematical study of blood flow. Based on many pilot studies, CFD is poised to have an increasingly powerful role in the care of patients with CVD in the next decade, by allowing a more refined understanding of the hemodynamics of both acquired CVD due to atherosclerosis and CHD. Continued partnerships between clinician-scientists and engineers are essential to the successful achievement of this goal. Only with such collaborations will the complex process of patient-specific modeling be streamlined and successfully integrated into clinical decision making to optimize medical and interventional therapies for cardiovascular disease.

Acknowledgements

The authors would like to acknowledge Mara Koffarnus for her assistance in manuscript preparation. The authors also acknowledge Mary Draney PhD, Frandics Chan MD, PhD, Ronak Dholakia PhD, Laura Ellwein PhD, David Wendell PhD, and Joseph Cava MD PhD for technical assistance with some of the parts of the listed CFD results.

Author details

Margaret M. Samyn[1*] and John F. LaDisa[2]

*Address all correspondence to: msamyn@chw.org

1 Medical College of Wisconsin, Pediatrics (Cardiology), Milwaukee, WI, USA

2 Marquette University, Biomedical Engineering, Milwaukee, WI, USA

References

[1] Mozaffarian D, Benjamin EJ, Go AS, Arnett DK, Blaha MJ, Cushman M, Das SR, de Ferranti S, Després J, Fullerton HJ, Howard VJ, Huffman MD, Isasi CR, Jiménez MC, Judd SE, Kissela BM, Lichtman JH, Lisabeth LD, Liu S, Mackey RH, Magid DJ, McGuire DK, Mohler ER, Moy CS, Muntner P, Mussolino ME, Nasir K, Neumar RW, Nichol G, Palaniappan L, Pandey DK, Reeves MJ, Rodriguez CJ, Rosamond W, Sorlie PD, Stein J, Towfighi A, Turan TN, Virani SS, Woo D, Yeh RW, Turner MB. Heart disease and stroke

statistics—2016 update: a report from the American Heart Association. Circulation. 2016;133:e38–e360. DOI: 10.1161/CIR.0000000000000350.

[2] 2012 European Cardiovascular Disease Statistics [Internet]. 2016. Available from: http://www.escardio.org/The-ESC/Initiatives/EuroHeart/2012-European-Cardiovascular-Disease-Statistics [Accessed: 4/7/2016].

[3] Marelli A, Gilboa S, Devine O, Kucik J, lonescu-lttu R, Oster M, Riehle-Colarusso T, Correa A, Jenkins K. Estimating the congenital heart disease population in the United States in 2010—what are the numbers? Journal of the American College of Cardiology. 2012;59:E787–E787.

[4] Wolinsky H, Glagov S. Comparison of abdominal and thoracic aortic medial structure in mammals. Circulation Research. 1969;25:677–686. DOI: 10.1161/01.RES.25.6.677.

[5] Xu CP, Glagov S, Zatina MA, Zarins CK. Hypertension sustains plaque progression despite reduction of hypercholesterolemia. Hypertension. 1991;18:123–129. DOI: 10.1161/01.HYP.18.2.123.

[6] Liu SQ, Fung YC. Relationship between hypertension, hypertrophy, and opening angle of zero-stress state of arteries following aortic constriction. Journal of Biomechanical Engineering. 1989;111:325–335. DOI: 10.1115/1.3168386.

[7] Kleinstreuer C, Hyun S, Buchanan JR Jr, Longest PW, Archie JP Jr, Truskey GA. Hemodynamic parameters and early intimal thickening in branching blood vessels. Critical Reviews in Biomedical Engineering. 2001;29:1–64.

[8] Ku DN, Giddens DP, Zarins CK, Glagov S. Pulsatile flow and atherosclerosis in the human carotid bifurcation. Positive Correlation between plaque location and low oscillating shear stress. Arteriosclerosis, Thrombosis, and Vascular Biology. 1985;5:293–302. DOI: 10.1161/01.ATV.5.3.293.

[9] Lehoux SS, Tronc F, Tedgui A. Mechanisms of blood flow-induced vascular enlargement. Biorheology. 2002;39:319–324.

[10] Malek AM, Alper SL, Izumo S. Hemodynamic shear stress and its role in atherosclerosis. Journal of the American Medical Association. 1999;282:2035–2042.

[11] Moore JE, Xu C, Glagov S, Zarins CK, Ku DN. Fluid wall shear stress measurements in a model of the human abdominal aorta: oscillatory behavior and relationship to atherosclerosis. Atherosclerosis. 1994;110:225–240. DOI: 10.1016/0021-9150(94)90207-0.

[12] Ojha M. Spatial and temporal variations of wall shear stress within an end-to-side arterial anastomosis model. Journal of Biomechanics. 1993;26:1377–1388. DOI: 10.1016/0021-9290(93)90089-W.

[13] De Nevers N. Fluid Mechanics for Chemical Engineers. 3rd ed. Boston: McGraw-Hill Higher Education; 2005. 632 p.

[14] LaDisa JFJ, Dholakia RJ, Figueroa CA, Vignon-Clementel IE, Chan FP, Samyn MM, Cava JR, Taylor CA, Feinstein JA. Computational simulations demonstrate altered wall shear

stress in aortic coarctation patients treated by resection with end-to-end anastomosis. Congenital Heart Disease. 2011;6:432–443. DOI: 10.1111/j.1747-0803.2011.00553.x.

[15] Müller J, Sahni O, Li X, Jansen KE, Shephard MS, Taylor CA. Anisotropic adaptive finite element method for modelling blood flow. Computer Methods in Biomechanics and Biomedical Engineering. 2005;8:295–305. DOI: 10.1080/10255840500264742.

[16] Sahni O, Müller J, Jansen KE, Shephard MS, Taylor CA. Efficient anisotropic adaptive discretization of the cardiovascular system. Computer Methods in Applied Mechanics and Engineering. 2006;195:5634–5655. DOI: 10.1016/j.cma.2005.10.018.

[17] Nichols W. McDonald's Blood Flow in Arteries: Theoretical, Experimental and Clinical Principles. 5th ed. Boca Raton, FL: CRC Press; 2005. 570 p.

[18] Sankaran S, Esmaily Moghadam M, Kahn AM, Tseng EE, Guccione JM, Marsden AL. Patient-specific multiscale modeling of blood flow for coronary artery bypass graft surgery. Annals of Biomedical Engineering. 2012;40:2228–2242. DOI: 10.1007/s10439-012-0579-3.

[19] Figueroa CA, Vignon-Clementel IE, Jansen KE, Hughes TJR, Taylor CA. A coupled momentum method for modeling blood flow in three-dimensional deformable arteries. Computer Methods in Applied Mechanics and Engineering. 2006;195:5685–5706. DOI: 10.1016/j.cma.2005.11.011.

[20] Lotz J, Meier C, Leppert A, Galanski M. Cardiovascular flow measurement with phase-contrast MR imaging: basic facts and implementation. RadioGraphics. 2002;22:651–671.

[21] Stergiopulos NN, Meister JJ, Westerfhoff N. Simple and accurate way for estimating total and segmental arterial compliance: the pulse pressure method. Annals of Biomedical Engineering. 1994;22:392–397.

[22] Stergiopulos NS. Use of pulse pressure method for estimating total arterial compliance in vivo. American Journal of Physiology—Heart and Circulatory Physiology. 1999;276:H424–H428.

[23] Samyn M, Dholakia R, Wang H, Co-Vu J, Yan K, Widlansky M, LaDisa J, Simpson P, Alemzadeh R. Cardiovascular magnetic resonance imaging-based computational fluid dynamics/fluid structure interaction pilot study to detect early vascular changes in pediatric patients with Type 1 diabetes. Pediatric Cardiology. 2015;36:851–861. DOI: 10.1007/s00246-014-1071-7.

[24] Kilner PJ, Yang GZ, Mohiaddin RH, Firmin DN, Longmore DB. Helical and retrograde secondary flow patterns in the aortic arch studied by three-directional magnetic resonance velocity mapping. Circulation. 1993;88:2235–2247.

[25] Liu X, Sun A, Fan Y, Deng X. Physiological significance of helical flow in the arterial system and its potential clinical applications. Annals of Biomedical Engineering. 2015;43:3–15. DOI: 10.1007/s10439-014-1097-2.

[26] Niezen RA, Doornbos J, van der Wall EE, de Roos A. Measurement of aortic and pulmonary flow with MRI at rest and during physical exercise. Journal of Computer Assisted Tomography. 1998;22:194–201.

[27] Weber TF, von Tengg-Kobligk H, Kopp-Schneider A, Ley-Zaporozhan J, Kauczor H, Ley S. High-Resolution phase-contrast MRI of aortic and pulmonary blood flow during rest and physical exercise using a MRI compatible bicycle ergometer. European Journal of Radiology. 2011;80:103–108. DOI: 10.1016/j.ejrad.2010.06.045.

[28] Pedersen EM, Kozerke S, Ringgaard S, Scheidegger MB, Boesiger P. Quantitative abdominal aortic flow measurements at controlled levels of ergometer exercise. Magnetic Resonance Imaging. 1999;17:489–494. DOI: 10.1016/S0730-725X(98)00209-4.

[29] Steeden JA, Atkinson D, Taylor AM, Muthurangu V. Assessing vascular response to exercise using a combination of real-time spiral phase contrast MR and noninvasive blood pressure measurements. Journal of Magnetic Resonance Imaging. 2010;31:997–1003. DOI: 10.1002/jmri.22105.

[30] Sampath S, Derbyshire JA, Ledesma-Carbayo MJ, McVeigh ER. Imaging left ventricular tissue mechanics and hemodynamics during supine bicycle exercise using a combined tagging and phase-contrast MRI pulse sequence. Magnetic Resonance in Medicine. 2011;65:51–59. DOI: 10.1002/mrm.22668.

[31] Taylor CA, Cheng CP, Espinosa LA, Tang BT, Parker D, Herfkens RJ. In vivo quantification of blood flow and wall shear stress in the human abdominal aorta during lower limb exercise. Annals of Biomedical Engineering. 30:402–408. DOI: 10.1114/1.1476016.

[32] Cheng CP, Schwandt DF, Topp EL, Anderson JH, Herfkens RJ, Taylor CA. Dynamic exercise imaging with an MR-compatible stationary cycle within the general electric open magnet. Magnetic Resonance in Medicine. 2003;49:581–585. DOI: 10.1002/mrm.10364.

[33] Cheng CP, Herfkens RJ, Lightner AL, Taylor CA, Feinstein JA. Blood flow conditions in the proximal pulmonary arteries and vena cavae: healthy children during upright cycling exercise. American Journal of Physiology–Heart and Circulatory Physiology. 2004;287:H921–H926. DOI: 10.1152/ajpheart.00022.2004.

[34] Kim HJ, Vignon-Clementel I, Figueroa CA, LaDisa JF, Jansen KE, Feinstein JA, Taylor CA. On coupling a lumped parameter heart model and a three-dimensional finite element aorta model. Annals of Biomedical Engineering. 2009;37:2153–2169. DOI: 10.1007/s10439-009-9760-8.

[35] LaDisa JFJ, Figueroa CA, Vignon-Clementel I, Kim HJ, Xiao N, Ellwein LM, Chan FP, Feinstein JA, Taylor CA. Computational simulations for aortic coarctation: representative results from a sampling of patients. Journal of Biomechanical Engineering. 2011;133:091008–091008.

[36] Ellwein L, Samyn MM, Danduran M, Schindler-Ivens S, Liebham S, LaDisa Jr. JF. Toward translating near-infrared spectroscopy oxygen saturation data for the non-

invasive predication of spatial and temporal hemodynamics during exercise. Biomechanics and Modeling in Mechanobiology. 2016 [Epub ahead of print].

[37] Frydrychowicz A, Stalder AF, Russe MF, Bock J, Bauer S, Harloff A, Berger A, Langer M, Hennig J, Markl M. Three-dimensional analysis of segmental wall shear stress in the aorta by flow-sensitive four-dimensional-MRI. Journal of Magnetic Resonance Imaging. 2009;30:77–84. DOI: 10.1002/jmri.21790.

[38] Wentzel JJ, Corti R, Fayad ZA, Wisdom P, Macaluso F, Winkelman MO, Fuster V, Badimon JJ. Does shear stress modulate both plaque progression and regression in the thoracic aorta?: Human study using serial magnetic resonance imaging. Journal of the American College of Cardiology. 2005;45:846–854. DOI: 10.1016/j.jacc.2004.12.026.

[39] LaDisa JF, Olson LE, Guler I, Hettrick DA, Kersten JR, Warltier DC, Pagel PS. Circumferential vascular deformation after stent implantation alters wall shear stress evaluated with time-dependent 3D computational fluid dynamics models. Journal of Applied Physiology. 2005;98:947–957. DOI: 10.1152/japplphysiol.00872.2004.

[40] White CR, Haidekker M, Bao X, Frangos JA. Temporal gradients in shear, but not spatial gradients, stimulate endothelial cell proliferation. Circulation. 2001;103:2508–2513.

[41] Hope MD, Meadows AK, Hope TA, Ordovas KG, Saloner D, Reddy GP, Alley MT, Higgins CB. Clinical evaluation of aortic coarctation with 4D flow MR imaging. Journal of Magnetic Resonance Imaging. 2010;31:711–718. DOI: 10.1002/jmri.22083.

[42] Markl M, Kilner PJ, Ebbers T. Comprehensive 4D velocity mapping of the heart and great vessels by cardiovascular magnetic resonance. Journal of Cardiovascular Magnetic Resonance. 2011;13:1–22. DOI: 10.1186/1532-429X-13-7.

[43] Barker AJ, Markl M, Bürk J, Lorenz R, Bock J, Bauer S, Schulz-Menger J, von Knobelsdorff-Brenkenhoff F. Bicuspid aortic valve is associated with altered wall shear stress in the ascending aorta. Circulation: Cardiovascular Imaging. 2012;5:457–466.

[44] Bieging ET, Frydrychowicz A, Wentland A, Landgraf BR, Johnson KM, Wieben O, François CJ. In vivo three-dimensional MR wall shear stress estimation in ascending aortic dilatation. Journal of Magnetic Resonance Imaging. 2011;33:589–597. DOI: 10.1002/jmri.22485.

[45] van Ooij P, Potters WV, Nederveen AJ, Allen BD, Collins J, Carr J, Malaisrie SC, Markl M, Barker AJ. A methodology to detect abnormal relative wall shear stress on the full surface of the thoracic aorta using four-dimensional flow MRI. Magnetic Resonance in Medicine. 2015;73:1216–1227. DOI: 10.1002/mrm.25224.

[46] Wendell DC, Samyn MM, Cava JR, Krolikowski MM, LaDisa JF. The impact of cardiac motion on aortic valve flow used in computational simulations of the thoracic aorta. Journal of Biomechanical Engineering. 2016;138(9) DOI: 10.1115/1.4033964.

[47] Morris PD, Narracott A, von Tengg-Kobligk H, Silva Soto DA, Hsiao S, Lungu A, Evans P, Bressloff NW, Lawford PV, Hose DR, Gunn JP. Computational fluid dynamics

modelling in cardiovascular medicine. Heart. 2016;102:18–28. DOI: 10.1136/heartjnl-2015-308044.

[48] Libby P. The vascular biology of atherosclerosis. In: Mann DL, Zipes DP, Libby P, Bonow RO, editors. Braunwald's Heart Disease: A Textbook of Cardiovascular Medicine. 10th ed. Philadelphia, PA: Elsevier Health Sciences; 2014. p. 873–890.

[49] Berenson GS, Srnivasan SR. Cardiovascular risk factors in youth with implications for aging: the bogalusa heart study. Neurobiology of Aging. 2005;26:303–307. DOI: 10.1016/j.neurobiolaging.2004.05.009.

[50] Juonala M, Magnussen CG, Venn A, Dwyer T, Burns TL, Davis PH, Chen W, Srinivasan SR, Daniels SR, Kähönen M, Laitinen T, Taittonen L, Berenson GS, Viikari JSA, Raitakari OT. Influence of age on associations between childhood risk factors and carotid intima-media thickness in adulthood: The Cardiovascular Risk in Young Finns Study, the Childhood Determinants of Adult Health Study, the Bogalusa Heart Study, and the Muscatine Study for the International Childhood Cardiovascular Cohort (i3C) Consortium. Circulation. 2010;122:2514–2520. DOI: 10.1161/CIRCULATIONAHA.110.966465.

[51] Tracy RE, Newman WPI, Wattigney WA, Berenson GS. Risk factors and atherosclerosis in youth autopsy findings of the Bogalusa Heart Study. American Journal of the Medical Sciences. 1995;310:S42.

[52] Glagov S, Weisenberg E, Zarins CK, Stankunavicius R, Kolettis GJ. Compensatory enlargement of human atherosclerotic coronary arteries. New England Journal of Medicine. 1987;316:1371–1375. DOI: 10.1056/NEJM198705283162204.

[53] Katranas SA, Antoniadis AP, Kelekis AL, Giannoglou GD. Insights on atherosclerosis by non-invasive assessment of wall stress and arterial morphology along the length of human coronary plaques. The International Journal of Cardiovascular Imaging. 2015;31:1627–1633. DOI: 10.1007/s10554-015-0736-5.

[54] LaDisa JF, Bowers M, Harmann L, Prost R, Doppalapudi AV, Mohyuddin T, Zaidat O, Migrino RQ. Time-efficient patient-specific quantification of regional carotid artery fluid dynamics and spatial correlation with plaque burden. Medical Physics. 2010;37:784–792. DOI: 10.1118/1.3292631.

[55] Babar GS, Zidan H, Widlansky ME, Das E, Hoffmann RG, Daoud M, Alemzadeh R. Impaired endothelial function in preadolescent children with Type 1 DIABETES. Diabetes Care. 2011;34:681–685. DOI: 10.2337/dc10-2134.

[56] Pasterkamp G, Galis ZS, de Kleijn DPV. Expansive arterial remodeling: location, location, location. Arteriosclerosis, Thrombosis, and Vascular Biology. 2004;24:650–657. DOI: 10.1161/01.ATV.0000120376.09047.fe.

[57] Brown JW, Ruzmetov M, Hoyer MH, Rodefeld MD, Turrentine MW. Recurrent coarctation: is surgical repair of recurrent coarctation of the aorta safe and effective?

The Annals of Thoracic Surgery. 2009;88:1923–1931. DOI: 10.1016/j.athoracsur.2009.07.024.

[58] Kron IL, Flanagan TL, Rheuban KS, Carpenter MA, Gutgesell HPJ, Blackbourne LH, Nolan SP. Incidence and risk of reintervention after coarctation repair. Annals of Thoracic Surgery. 1990;49:920–926.

[59] Kavey RW, Allada V, Daniels SR, Hayman LL, McCrindle BW, Newburger JW, Parekh RS, Steinberger J. Cardiovascular risk reduction in high-risk pediatric patients: a scientific statement from the American Heart Association Expert Panel on Population and Prevention Science; the Councils on Cardiovascular Disease in the Young, Epidemiology and Prevention, Nutrition, Physical Activity and Metabolism, High Blood Pressure Research, Cardiovascular Nursing, and the Kidney in Heart Disease; and the Interdisciplinary Working Group on Quality of Care and Outcomes Research: Endorsed by the American Academy of Pediatrics. Circulation. 2006;114:2710–2738. DOI: 10.1161/CIRCULATIONAHA.106.179568.

[60] Dholakia, Ronak J. Numerical modeling of hemodynamics in the thoracic aorta and alterations by dacron patch treatment of aortic coarctation [Thesis]. Milwaukee: Marquette University; 2009.

[61] Wendell DC, Samyn MM, Cava JR, Ellwein LM, Krolikowski MM, Gandy KL, Pelech AN, Shadden SC, LaDisa Jr. JF. Including aortic valve morphology in computational fluid dynamics simulations: initial findings and application to aortic coarctation. Medical Engineering & Physics. 2013;35:723–735. DOI: 10.1016/j.medengphy.2012.07.015.

[62] Camarda JA, Earing MG, Dholakia RJ, Wang H, Kwon S, LaDisa JF, Samyn MM. Biophysical properties of the aorta in patients with marfan syndrome and related connective tissue disorders: evaluation with MRI and computational fluid dynamics modeling. Journal of Cardiovascular Magnetic Resonance. 2011;13:P219.

[63] Golesworthy T, Lampérth M, Mohiaddin R, Pepper J, Thornton W, Treasure T. The tailor of gloucester: a jacket for the Marfan's aorta. The Lancet. 364:1582. DOI: 10.1016/S0140-6736(04)17308-X.

[64] Singh SD, Xu XY, Wood NB, Pepper JR, Izgi C, Treasure T, Mohiaddin RH. Aortic flow patterns before and after personalised external aortic root support implantation in Marfan patients. Journal of Biomechanics. 2016;49:100–111. DOI: 10.1016/j.jbiomech.2015.11.040.

[65] Johnson TR, Samyn MM, Sena L. Cardiac CT and MR evaluation of the adult Fontan patient. In: Saremi F, editor. Cardiac CT and MR for Adult Congenital Heart Disease New York: Springer Science & Business Media; 2013. p. 481–498. DOI: 10.1007/978-1-4614-8875-0.

[66] Superior Cavopulmonary Anastomosis: The Hemi-Fontan and Bidirectional Glenn [Internet]. 2016. Available from: http://www.ctsnet.org/article/superior-cavopulmonary-anastomosis-hemi-fontan-and-bidirectional-glenn [Accessed: 4/12/2016].

[67] Modified Fontan [Internet]. 2016. Available from: http://www.ctsnet.org/article/modified-fontan [Accessed: 4/12/2016].

[68] Tang E, Yoganathan AP. Optimizing hepatic flow distribution with the Fontan Y-Graft: lessons from computational simulations. The Journal of Thoracic and Cardiovascular Surgery. 2015;149:255–256. DOI: 10.1016/j.jtcvs.2014.09.094.

[69] Pike NA, Vricella LA, Feinstein JA, Black MD, Reitz BA. Regression of severe pulmonary arteriovenous malformations after Fontan revision and "hepatic factor" rerouting. The Annals of Thoracic Surgery. 2004;78:697–699. DOI: 10.1016/j.athoracsur.2004.02.003.

[70] Srivastava D, Preminger T, Lock JE, Mandell V, Keane JF, Mayer JE, Kozakewich H, Spevak PJ. Hepatic venous blood and the development of pulmonary arteriovenous malformations in congenital heart disease. Circulation. 1995;92:1217–1222. DOI: 10.1161/01.CIR.92.5.1217.

[71] Knight WB, Mee RBB. A cure for pulmonary arteriovenous fistulas? The Annals of Thoracic Surgery. 1995;59:999–1001. DOI: 10.1016/0003-4975(94)00735-P.

[72] Vettukattil JJ. Pathogenesis of pulmonary arteriovenous malformations: role of hepatopulmonary interactions. Heart. 2002;88:561–563. DOI: 10.1136/heart.88.6.561.

[73] Migliavacca F, Pennati G, Dubini G, Fumero R, Pietrabissa R, Urcelay G, Bove E, Hsia T, deLeval M. Modeling of the Norwood circulation: effects of shunt size, vascular resistances, and heart rate. American Journal of Physiology—Heart and Circulatory Physiology. 2001;280:H2076–2086.

[74] Biglino G, Giardini A, Hsia T, Figliola R, Taylor AM, Schievano S. Modelling single ventricle physiology: review of engineering tools to study first stage palliation of hypoplastic left heart syndrome. Frontiers in Pediatrics. 2013;1. DOI: 10.3389/fped.2013.00031.

[75] Pennati G, Corsini C, Hsia T, Migliavacca F. computational fluid dynamics models and congenital heart diseases. Frontiers in Pediatrics. 2013;1(4). DOI: 10.3389/fped.2013.00004.

[76] Troianowski G, Taylor CA, Feinstein JA, Vignon-Clementel I. Three-dimensional simulations in glenn patients: clinically based boundary conditions, hemodynamic results and sensitivity to input data. Journal of Biomechanical Engineering. 2011;133:111006–111006. DOI: 10.1115/1.4005377.

[77] Sun Q, Wan D, Liu J, Hong H, Liu Y, Zhu M. Patient-specific computational fluid dynamic simulation of a bilateral bidirectional glenn connection. Medical & Biological Engineering & Computing. 2008;46:1153–1159. DOI: 10.1007/s11517-008-0376-1.

[78] de Zélicourt DA, Pekkan K, Parks J, Kanter K, Fogel M, Yoganathan AP. Flow Study of an extracardiac connection with persistent left superior vena cava. The Journal of Thoracic and Cardiovascular Surgery. 2006;131:785–791. DOI: 10.1016/j.jtcvs.2005.11.031.

[79] de Leval MR, Dubini G, Migliavacca F, Jalali H, Camporini G, Redington A, Pietrabissa R. Use of Computational fluid dynamics in the design of surgical procedures: application to the study of competitive flows in cavopulmonary connections. The Journal of Thoracic and Cardiovascular Surgery. 1996;111:502–513. DOI: 10.1016/S0022-5223(96)70302-1.

[80] de Leval MR, Kilner PJ, Gewillig M, Bull C. Total cavopulmonary connection: a logical alternative to atriopulmonary connection for complex fontan operations. Experimental Studies and Early Clinical Experience. Journal of Thoracic and Cardiovascular Surgery. 1988;96:682–95.

[81] Bove EL, de Leval MR, Migliavacca F, Balossino R, Dubini G. Toward optimal hemodynamics: computer modeling of the fontan circuit. Pediatric Cardiology. 2007;28:477–481. DOI: 10.1007/s00246-007-9009-y".

[82] de Zélicourt DA, Haggerty CM, Sundareswaran KS, Whited BS, Rossignac JR, Kanter KR, Gaynor JW, Spray TL, Sotiropoulos F, Fogel MA, Yoganathan AP. Individualized computer-based surgical planning to address pulmonary arteriovenous malformations in patients with a single ventricle with an interrupted inferior vena cava and azygous continuation. The Journal of Thoracic and Cardiovascular Surgery. 2011;141:1170–1177. DOI: 10.1016/j.jtcvs.2010.11.032.

[83] Haggerty CM, de Zélicourt DA, Restrepo M, Rossignac J, Spray TL, Kanter KR, Fogel MA, Yoganathan AP. Comparing pre- and post-operative Fontan hemodynamic simulations: implications for the reliability of surgical planning. Annals of Biomedical Engineering. 2012;40:2639–2651. DOI: 10.1007/s10439-012-0614-4.

[84] Marsden AL, Bernstein AJ, Reddy VM, Shadden SC, Spilker RL, Chan FP, Taylor CA, Feinstein JA. Evaluation of a novel Y-shaped extracardiac Fontan Baffle using computational fluid dynamics. The Journal of Thoracic and Cardiovascular Surgery. 2009;137:394–403.e2. DOI: 10.1016/j.jtcvs.2008.06.043.

[85] Soerensen DD, Pekkan K, de Zélicourt D, Sharma S, Kanter K, Fogel M, Yoganathan AP. Introduction of a new optimized total cavopulmonary connection. The Annals of Thoracic Surgery. 2007;83:2182–2190. DOI: 10.1016/j.athoracsur.2006.12.079.

[86] Yang W, Vignon-Clementel IE, Troianowski G, Reddy VM, Feinstein JA, Marsden AL. Hepatic blood flow distribution and performance in conventional and novel Y-graft Fontan geometries: a case series computational fluid dynamics study. The Journal of Thoracic and Cardiovascular Surgery. 2012;143:1086–1097. DOI: 10.1016/j.jtcvs.2011.06.042.

[87] Samyn MM, Kwon EN, Gorentz JS, Yan K, Danduran MJ, Cava JR, Simpson PM, Frommelt PC, Tweddell JS. Restrictive versus nonrestrictive physiology following

repair of Tetralogy of Fallot: is there a difference? Journal of the American Society of Echocardiography. 2013;26:746–755. DOI: 10.1016/j.echo.2013.03.019.

[88] Kilner PJ, Balossino R, Dubini G, Babu-Narayan SV, Taylor AM, Pennati G, Migliavacca F. Pulmonary regurgitation: the effects of varying pulmonary artery compliance, and of increased resistance proximal or distal to the compliance. International Journal of Cardiology. 2009;133:157–166. DOI: 10.1016/j.ijcard.2008.06.078.

[89] Samyn MM, Powell AJ, Garg R, Sena L, Geva T. Range of ventricular dimensions and function by steady-state free precession cine MRI in repaired Tetralogy of Fallot: right ventricular outflow tract patch vs. conduit repair. Journal of Magnetic Resonance Imaging. 2007;26:934–940.

[90] Geva T. Indications for pulmonary valve replacement in repaired Tetralogy of Fallot: the quest continues. Circulation. 2013;128:1855–1857. DOI: 10.1161/CIRCULATIONA-HA.113.005878.

[91] Chern M, Wu M, Wang H. Numerical investigation of regurgitation phenomena in pulmonary arteries of Tetralogy of Fallot patients after repair. Journal of Biomechanics. 2008;41:3002–3009. DOI: 10.1016/j.jbiomech.2008.07.017.

[92] Guibert R, McLeod K, Caiazzo A, Mansi T, Fernández MA, Sermesant M, Pennec X, Vignon-Clementel IE, Boudjemline Y, Gerbeau J. Group-wise construction of reduced models for understanding and characterization of pulmonary blood flows from medical images. Medical Image Analysis. 2014;18:63–82. DOI: 10.1016/j.media.2013.09.003.

[93] Chern M, Wu M, Her S. Numerical study for blood flow in pulmonary arteries after repair of Tetralogy of Fallot. Computational and Mathematical Methods in Medicine 2012;198108:04/13/2016 DOI: 10.1155/2012/198108.

[94] Rao AS, Menon PG. Presurgical planning using image-based in silico anatomical and functional characterization of Tetralogy of Fallot with associated anomalies. Interactive Cardiovascular and Thoracic Surgery. 2015;20:149–156. DOI: 10.1093/icvts/ivu368.

[95] Caiazzo A, Guibert R, Vignon-Clementel I. A reduced-order modeling for efficient design study of artificial valve in enlarged ventricular outflow tracts. Computer Methods in Biomechanics and Biomedical Engineering. 2016;19(12):1314–1318. DOI: 10.1080/10255842.2015.1133811.

Chapter 4

Application of Spatial Bayesian Hierarchical Models to fMRI Data

Kuo-Jung Lee

Additional information is available at the end of the chapter

http://dx.doi.org/10.5772/64823

Abstract

Bayesian modelling has attracted great interest in cognitive science and offered a flexible and interpretable way to study cognitive processes using functional magnetic resonance imaging data. In this chapter, a spatial Bayesian hierarchical model is applied to an event-related fMRI study of cognitive control using the Simon test. We consider a sparse spatial generalized linear mixed-effects model to capture the spatial dependence among activated voxels and temporal parameters and to benefit computationally by reducing dimensionality. We demonstrate that the proposed model has the capability of identification of the brain areas related to cognitive tasks. Moreover, the reduction in the false positive rate is observed in the simulation study, and the relevant brain regions involved in processing cognitive control are clearly detected in a real-life fMRI example.

Keywords: Bayesian, functional magnetic resonance imaging, Markov chain Monte Carlo, spatial generalized linear mixed-effects model

1. Introduction

Functional magnetic resonance imaging (fMRI) has increasingly become an important and popular modality that allows researchers to investigate brain activity resulting from a particular stimulus [1]. In an fMRI experiment, a subject is asked to perform a task by responding to a series of stimuli that may involve a motor, sensory or cognitive task, then the MR machine records the changes in the blood oxygen level dependent (BOLD) of the brain across different time points, resulting in three-dimensional fMRI time-series images. Numerous statistical models have been proposed to allow researchers to detect localized regions activated during a task, to describe the networks required for a particular brain function or to assess physical characteristics elicited by cognitive processes in the brain. However, the growth in the complexity, the significant size and the hierarchical structure of fMRI data make it difficult to comprise a fully efficient computationally feasible statistical model to accurately explain the temporal and spatial characteristics of the data.

The standard approach used on fMRI data is known as statistical parametric mapping (SPM) [2], which applied either a voxel-wise t-test or F-test statistics. In order to obtain an activation map of the brain, the next step is to threshold the test statistics at a given overall error rate that leads to a major multiplicity problem. The most common way of solving this problem is to use Gaussian random field theory [3]. This technique is based on the assumption of a stationary Gaussian random field, which may not be satisfied in fMRI settings. Another limitation is that most current methods ignore at least one of the spatial or temporal relationships between observations. Ignoring either spatial or temporal correlations in the model leads to seriously biased conclusions [4].

This article introduces a novel Bayesian modelling approach to fMRI data analysis. Bayesian approaches have great potential in applications because they allow a flexible modelling of spatial and temporal correlations in data [5]. We consider a Bayesian spatiotemporal model in a computationally feasible manner to detect brain regions that are activated by the external stimulus in fMRI. Accurate and powerful single-subject task-related activation models are required in order to develop effective imaging biomarkers, which constitutes the primary scientific problem. Moreover, the Bayesian paradigm provides an attractive inferential framework that can directly incorporate the physical characteristics of an experiment. Our goal is to put forward a model and inferential framework by which to investigate task-specific changes in the BOLD signal. Clearly, the model must account for the spatial relationships between the voxels, but there are other possible sources of variation that should not be ignored. Ultimately, we develop a hierarchical Bayesian model, which not only takes into account the spatiotemporal and temporal drift relationships in the data under consideration, but also easily investigates the role of specific regions that integrate brain activity to coordinate cognition and behaviour.

The applied Bayesian hierarchical approach contains several characteristics [4, 6]. Latent binary variables are introduced to indicate activation/inactivation of voxels. The spatial generalized linear mixed model (SGLMM) [7, 8] is considered to capture the spatial dependence of the latent binary variables. In addition, the autoregression (AR) model is used to model the temporal dependence of signal changes. Several studies have found that spatial dependence also appears in the temporal parameters in AR models [4, 9]. Thus, neglecting the spatial dependence of temporal correlations moderates the computational intensity, but the simplification may produce a biased estimation of the temporal coefficients and consequently may result in the spurious detection of brain activities [10]. Therefore, we also consider the spatial linear mixed-effects model to spatially regularize the AR parameters.

In fMRI data, the posterior inferences are based on the estimations of parameters; however, the posterior distribution is typically extremely large, and is unavailable in analytic form. Hence, we employ Markov chain Monte Carlo (MCMC) [11] sampling techniques that combine Metropolis-Hastings [12] schemes to generate samples from the posterior distribution for the purpose of performing inferential tasks. To reduce the computational burden and accelerate the sampling procedure, we parcel the brain so that sampling procedures can be performed in parallel. In addition, prior information on activation in the form of spatially informative variables, e.g. the grey and white areas of the brain, can be incorporated into the model.

2. Statistical modelling

In this section, we introduce the proposed statistical model in the analysis of fMRI data. To make inferences about task-related change in underlying neuronal activity, a general linear model is used to model BOLD signal changes for each voxel. In addition to the essential temporal dependence of BOLD signals in a voxel itself, the BOLD signal changes show spatially contiguous and locally homogenous among voxels [11]. Shmuel et al. [13] in the visual fMRI study have demonstrated BOLD response seems to be well approximated by separable spatiotemporal model. Thus, for computational convenience, we consider a Bayesian separable spatiotemporal model for BODL signal changes to simultaneously account for the temporal dependence in nearby time points and spatial dependence in local neighbouring voxels.

Let $y_v=(y_{v1}, \ldots, y_{vT})'$, be a $T \times 1$ column vector and denote the observed BOLD signals from a voxel $v=1, \ldots, V$ at time t, $t=1, \ldots, T$. Following [14], we model the BOLD response for a particular voxel v with a linear regression model defined as

$$y_v = X_v\beta_v + L_v\rho_v + \varepsilon_v; \quad \varepsilon_v \sim N_T(0, \sigma^2 I_T), \tag{1}$$

where X_v is the design matrix, each column of which consists of values obtained from an impulse stimulus function [15, 16] with respect to a task convolved with the hemodynamic response function (HRF); β_v, is a $p \times 1$ vector and corresponds to the effect of stimuli on the BOLD signal changes. The temporal correlation is modelled by ρ_v, being an $r \times 1$ autoregression coefficient vector, with L_v, a $T \times r$ matrix of lagged prediction errors [2, 14]. We assume that the error terms ϵ_v in (1) are independently normally distributed $N_T(0, \sigma^2 I_T)$ with a mean vector 0 of length T and a covariance matrix $\sigma^2 I_T$ across voxels, where I_T is a $T \times T$ identity matrix [14]. In the Bayesian framework, the parameters are hierarchically assigned and the corresponding priors are defined, including spatial prior being introduced to capture the spatial dependence of brain activities among voxels.

For the purpose of detecting the activation of a voxel, a vector of binary random variables $\gamma_v=(\gamma_{v1}, \ldots, \gamma_{vp})'$ is introduced to indicate whether the voxel v is in response to a sequence of input stimuli. The voxel v is considered active to the stimulus j if $\gamma_{vj}=1$ and, on the other hand, inactive if $\gamma_{vj}=0$. Given that γ_{vj}, we assume β_{vj} has a spike and slab mixture prior of two normal distributions [17] given by

$$\beta_{vj} \mid \gamma_{vj} \sim \gamma_{vj} N\left(0, c_{vj}^2 \tau_{vj}^2\right) + \left(1 - \gamma_{vj}\right) N\left(0, \tau_{vj}^2\right) \tag{2}$$

where $N(\mu, \sigma^2)$ is denoted as a normal distribution with a mean μ and a variance σ^2. In Eq. (2), we let c_{vj}^2 being fixed and assume τ_{vj}^2 to have an inverse gamma distribution $\mathcal{IG}\left(\frac{a_\tau}{2}, \frac{b_\tau}{2}\right)$ [4]. We consider that $X \sim \mathcal{G}(a, b)$ if the probability density function of X is defined by just below Eq. (3)

$$f(x|a,b) = \frac{b^a}{\Gamma(a)} x^{-a-1} e^{-b/x}, x > 0, \tag{3}$$

where $\Gamma(a) = \int_0^\infty y^{a-1} e^{-y} dy$. We set c_{vj}^2 to be large resulting in the nonzero estimate of β_{vj} so that the stimulus j is considered to activate the voxel v. As George et al. [17] suggested, c_{vj}^2 should be taken less than 10^4 to avoid the computational problems and we find that $c_{vj}^2 = 10$ is a reasonable choice in our simulation studies and real fMRI example.

Since the response at a particular voxel is likely to be consistent to the responses of neighbouring voxels, we apply SGLMM [7, 35] to capture the spatial relationship. We assume $\gamma_j = (\gamma_{1j}, \ldots, \gamma_{Vj})'$ are independently distributed in accordance to the Bernoulli distribution $\gamma_{vj} \mid \eta_{vj} \sim Ber(\eta_{vj})$ with a logistic link $\text{logit}(\eta_{vj}) = \alpha_{vj} + m'_v \phi_j$, where $\text{logit}(\eta_{vj}) = \ln\left(\frac{\eta_{vj}}{1 - \eta_{vj}}\right)$ and α_{vj} is a constant intended to incorporate the expert knowledge or anatomical information and ϕ_j is a vector of spatial random effects. The spatial dependence between the binary variables is implicitly captured by ϕ_j assuming to have

$$\phi_j | \kappa_j \sim N\left(0, \left(\kappa_j M' Q M\right)^{-1}\right), \tag{4}$$

where m'_v is v_{th} row of M, an $V \times q$ matrix consisting of multi-resolutional spatial basis vectors that are able to explain spatial variation sources. The columns of M, consist of the q principal eigenvectors with respect to the first q largest eigenvalues from the adjacency matrix A of voxels, an $V \times V$ matrix with the $(v, s)_{\text{th}}$ element in Eq. (5), defined as

$$A(v,s) = \begin{cases} 0 & v = s \\ 1 & v \sim s \end{cases}, \tag{5}$$

where $v \sim s$ indicates s and v are neighbours. In the three-dimensional fMRI data analysis, a 26-adjacent neighbourhood is considered [8]. Typically, q is less than $V/2$ or equal to the number of eigenvalues greater than 0.05. This choice can reduce the dimensionality significantly but still maintains the spatial structure of the data. The graph Laplacian matrix $Q = \text{diag}(A\mathbf{1}) - A$ relates spatial basis vectors to represent the image data [18] and $\mathbf{1}$ is a $q \times 1$ column vector of ones. We assume a conjugate prior for the smoothing parameter given by

http://dx.doi.org/10.5772/64823

$$\kappa_j \sim \mathcal{G}\left(\frac{a_K}{2}, \frac{b_K}{2}\right). \tag{6}$$

To avoid generating artefactual spatial structure in the posterior distribution, [19] suggested $a_\kappa = 1$ and $b_\kappa = 4000$ in Eq. (6). We refer $X \sim \mathcal{G}(a, b)$ if the probability density function of X is defined in just below Eq. (7)

$$f(x|a,b) = \frac{1}{\Gamma(a) b^a} x^{a-1} e^{-x/b}, x > 0. \tag{7}$$

It is also found that the temporal correlations between voxels tend similar [4]. Such spatial dependence is modelled by a spatial linear mixed-effects model. For computational convenience and simplicity, we make a transformation of ρ_{vr} such that $\tilde{\rho}_{vr} = \log\frac{1+\rho_{vr}}{1-\rho_{vr}}$ and assume $\tilde{\rho}_{vr} \sim N(m'_v \varphi_r, \lambda_r^2)$. For the spatial random effect for the temporal parameter $\tilde{\rho}_s$ is assumed to be

$$\varphi_r | \omega_r \sim (0, (\omega_r M' Q M)^{-1}), \tag{8}$$

where φ_r is the spatial random effect for the rth order of the temporal parameters, and M and Q in Eq. (8) are the same as those listed in Eq. (4). Finally, we assume that $\omega_r \sim \mathcal{G}\left(\frac{a_\omega}{2}, \frac{b_\omega}{2}\right)$, $\lambda_r^2 \sim \mathcal{IG}\left(\frac{a_\lambda}{2}, \frac{b_\lambda}{2}\right)$ and $\sigma^2 \sim \mathcal{IG}\left(\frac{a_\sigma}{2}, \frac{b_\sigma}{2}\right)$. The values of a's and b's in the gamma or inverse gamma distributions are determined by the user to reflect the strength of one's prior belief before observing the data.

3. Posterior inference

To explore parallel computation, which allows us to substantially speed-up expensive operations in the MCMC iteration, we partition the brain into non-overlapping areas such as rectangular three-dimensional lattices or Brodmann areas. We then carry out the statistical model in Section 2 to analyse the partitioned data. In this chapter, for simplicity, we use Brodmann's map to parcel the brain into distinct regions before implementing the proposed model to the real fMRI data. In addition, separate regions divided by a data-drive segmentation procedure using functional clustering can be considered. Next, we introduce the likelihood function and the priors combining the parcellation procedure to form the posterior distribution for inference.

Suppose that a brain can be divided into G parcels, where the gth parcel contains V_g voxels, $g = 1, \ldots, G$ and where we denote the voxel-level parameters as $\theta_v = (\beta_v, \rho_v, \gamma_v, \sigma_v^2)$ and the parcel-level parameters as $\Theta_g = (\varphi, \kappa, \tau^2, \lambda^2, \phi, \omega)$. The posterior distribution is obtained by combining the priors $\pi(\theta_v, \Theta_g)$ and the likelihood $L(\theta_v \mid y_v)$, which are defined in Eqs. (9) and (10) as follows [8, 20]:

$$\pi(\theta_v, \Theta_g) = \prod_{v=1}^{V_g} \pi(\rho_v)\pi(\sigma_v^2)\pi(\beta_v \mid \gamma_v) \prod_{j=1}^{p} \pi(\gamma_j \mid \phi_j)\pi(\phi_j \mid \kappa_j)\pi(\kappa_j)\pi(\tau_j^2) \prod_{k=1}^{r} \pi(\lambda_k)\pi(\varphi_k \mid \omega_k)\pi(\omega_k) \tag{9}$$

and

$$L(\theta_v \mid y_v) = \left(\frac{1}{2\pi\sigma_v^2}\right)^{-T/2} \exp\left\{-\frac{(y_v - X_v\beta_v - L_v\rho_v)'(y_v - X_v\beta_v - L_v\rho_v)}{2\sigma_v^2}\right\}. \tag{10}$$

Due to the intractability of the posterior, Gibbs and Metropolis-Hastings updates [20, 34] are applied to sample the posterior distribution for estimation and inference of the model parameters.

The posterior quantities of interest are $P(\gamma_{vj}=1 \mid y)$ for the activation map and $E(\beta_{vj} \mid y)$ for the magnitude of the effect caused by the stimulus j on the BOLD signal changes for voxel v. They can be directly estimated based on MCMC samples by

$$\hat{P}(\gamma_{vj} = 1 \mid y) = \frac{1}{M}\sum_{m=1}^{M} \gamma_{vj}^{(m)} \text{ and } \hat{E}(\beta_{vj} \mid y) = \frac{1}{M}\sum_{m=1}^{M} \beta_{vj}^{(m)}, \tag{11}$$

where $\gamma_{vj}^{(m)}$ and $\beta_{vj}^{(m)}$ are the mth sample from a total M MCMC samples for γ_{vj} and β_{vj}, respectively. The distribution of $\hat{P}(\gamma_{vj}=1 \mid y)$ in a map provides a way to visually inspect brain regions with peak, high, low and practically no activation. In addition, $\hat{E}(\beta_{vj} \mid y)$ in Eq. (11) offers researchers to view the strength of response in the brain to the stimulus.

The construction of the binary activation map is obtained by thresholding the posterior probability of $\gamma_{vj}=1$. A threshold value c needs to be used in the detection of brain activity, that is, a voxel v is defined as active to a stimulus j if $\hat{P}(\gamma_{vj}=1 \mid y)>c$. However, threshold determination lacks agreement among investigators. Under certain conditions, a median selection criterion, $c=0.5$, results in the minimum prediction risk [21]. Smith et al. [6] and Lee et al. [4] defined a threshold by matching a Bayes factor approximation to a likelihood ratio test for activation such that $c=0.8722$ at a 5% level of significance. Additional to both, Kalus et al. [22] applied the false discovery rate (FDR) [23] to determine a threshold. In practice, it would be reasonable to construct activation maps for a grid of thresholds and to evaluate elicited results with neuroscience experts. In our experience, activation maps seem to be comparably robust against an exact choice of the threshold.

4. Simulation studies

We conduct stimulation studies to investigate the performance of the proposed model on the detection of brain activity. We measure the accuracy of the classification of voxels as either active/inactive and show the proposed model to be robust with regard to different spatial structures. Finally, we illustrate the implementation of the proposed model to a simulated fMRI data that mimics a study in face repetition effects in memory tests [24].

4.1. Benchmark example

Consider a 30×30 binary activation image γ_v, v 1, …, 900, generated independently from

$$\gamma_v \mid \eta_v \sim Ber(\eta_v), \tag{12}$$

where $\text{logit}(\eta_v) = \alpha_v + m'_v\phi$ and

$$\phi \mid \kappa \sim N\left(0, (\kappa M'QM)^{-1}\right). \tag{13}$$

We let $\alpha_v = 0$, $\kappa = 0.5$, where M is a 300×900 matrix whose columns are $q = 300$ principal eigenvectors of the adjacency matrix, A, for the image corresponding to the first $q = 300$ largest eigenvalues. Moreover, m'_v is the v_{th} row of M, and $Q = \text{diag}(A\mathbf{1}) - A$.

We consider an AR(1) temporal correlation between time points within voxels. For each voxel v, let $\tilde{\rho}_v = \log\frac{1+\rho_v}{1-\rho_v}$ and $\tilde{\rho}_v$ are generated from

$$\tilde{\rho}_v \sim N(m'_v\varphi, \lambda^2) \text{ and } \varphi \mid \omega \sim N(0, (\omega M'QM)^{-1}). \tag{14}$$

We let $\lambda^2 = 0.1$ and $\omega = 2$.

We consider a stimulus and the block and event-related designs with a total number of time points spanning 400 and repetition time (TR) equal to 2s. In the block design, the duration time is 20s. In the event-related design, the stimulus is randomly assigned. The stimulus function is convolved with a HRF modelled by a double gamma function [15] to create the design matrix

X_v. The stimulus functions and the corresponding design matrices for the block and event-related designs are shown in **Figure 1(a)** and **(b)**, respectively.

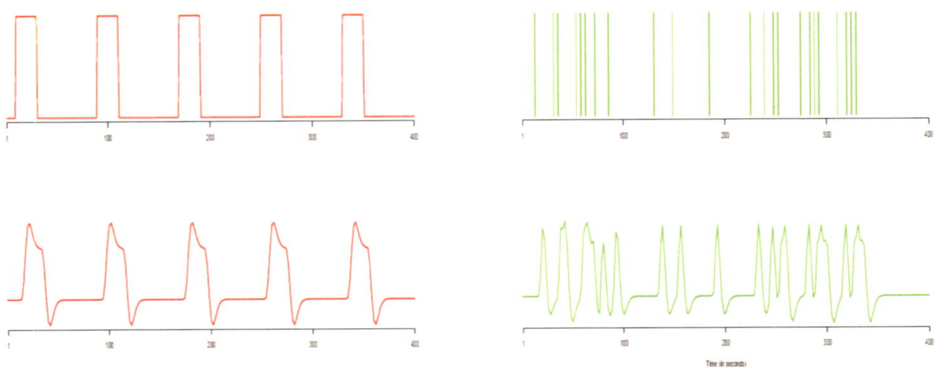

(a) Block design. (b) Event-related design.

Figure 1. The stimulus functions and the predicted BOLD signal changes used in the Benchmark example.

Given X_v, γ_v, ρ_v, the BOLD signal changes y_v are generated from a normal distribution with a covariance $\sigma_v^2 \Lambda_v$, where σ_v^2=1 and the $(u, v)_{\text{th}}$ element of Λ_v is $\rho^{|u-v|}$, and a mean of $X_v \beta_v$, where

$$\beta_v = \begin{cases} 3 & \text{if} \quad \gamma_v = 1; \\ 0 & \text{if} \quad \gamma_v = 0. \end{cases} \tag{15}$$

We then apply the proposed model to detect the activation areas, that is, to identify which voxel has γ_v=1. We ran MCMC chains with 100,000 iterations in order to ensure the largest Monte Carlo standard error (MCSE) [25] of all posterior probabilities of γ_v=1, less than 0.01.

We obtained posterior activation maps by setting the posterior probability threshold at 0.8722, that is, the voxel is categorized as active if $\hat{P}(\gamma_v = 1 \mid y) > 0.8722$, and it is categorized as inactive otherwise [26]. To measure the performance of our proposed model, we calculate the true classification rate (TCR), the true positive rate (TPR) and the false positive rate (FPR), which are defined as

$$\text{TCR} = \frac{\text{number of correctly classified voxels}}{\text{number of voxels}}; \tag{16}$$

$$\text{TPR} = \frac{\text{number of active voxels correctly claimed as active}}{\text{number of active voxels}}; \tag{17}$$

$$\text{FPR} = \frac{\text{number of inactive voxels correctly claimed as active}}{\text{number of inactive voxels}}. \tag{18}$$

Table 1 shows the proposed method performs well with regard to detecting the active voxels where only a small number of active voxels are falsely identified as inactive in both designs. Over 10 replications, the model with consideration of spatial dependence performs better on the detection of activations. Especially, FPR reduces around 50%.

(a)		
	Block design (%)	Event-related design (%)
TCR	92.44 (90.28–96.67)	91.12 (91.82–96.00)
TPR	99.97 (99.94–100)	99.97 (99.94–100)
FPR	6.98 (3.45–8.75)	6.54 (3.54–8.66)
(b)		
	Block design (%)	Event-related design (%)
TCR	96.33 (95.89–97.56)	95.78 (95.12–97.50)
TPR	99.99 (99.97–100)	99.99 (99.97–100)
FPR	3.42 (1.12–5.27)	3.22 (1.32–4.78)

The values within the parentheses are the range of different rates over 10 replications.

Table 1. The percentage of correct classification of voxels with a threshold at 0.8722 for considering the spatial dependence in (a) and without considering spatial dependence in (b) for temporal parameters in the model.

4.2. Structures with spatial dependence

To demonstrate that the proposed model is able to handle the different binary and temporal image spatial dependencies, we generate a dataset that is the same as the benchmark example in the paper of [27]. We create a 20×20 binary image as shown in **Figure 2(a)**, where the areas in red indicate that the voxels are active, and otherwise, they are not. Moreover, the values of ρs are generated from a uniform distribution between –0.3 and 0.3 for the non-active areas. However, we assign the fixed values –0.5, 0.5, and 0.75 to ρ in each active area, respectively, as shown in **Figure 2(b)**. This is designed to investigate the patterns of temporal dependencies within the different areas. Similar to the settings discussed in Section 3.1, we consider both block and event-related designs with one stimulus. First, β_v's generated from $U(2, 5)$ and σ_v^2 from $U(1, 3)$. The design matrix X_v and temporal correlation matrix Λ_v are defined to be the same as in Section 3.1. Given X_v, γ_v, ρ_v, β_v, and σ_v^2 the BOLD signal changes are generated from a normal distribution with a mean $X_v\beta_v$ and a covariance $\sigma_v^2\Lambda_v$. We carry out the proposed approach to detect the activation and estimate the parameters of interest. For ease of visualization of the results, we provide one of the estimated binary images without thresholding and the corresponding estimated image, as shown in **Figure 2(c)**. By visually inspecting estimated values of ρs in **Figure 2(d)** compared to the simulated ones in **Figure 2(b)**, we are confident that the spatial dependences also can be captured by the model.

After thresholding by a value determined by controlling FDR as 0.05, the accuracy of the classification of voxels measured by TCR is 99.25%, and the FPR is 4.84% with consideration of the spatial dependence of the temporal correlations over 10 replications. On the other hand, when the threshold is taken to be equal to 0.8722, TCR is 99.17% and FPR is 5.01%. Therefore, the proposed model can be applied to detect the activation of brain image data even for different spatial dependence structures.

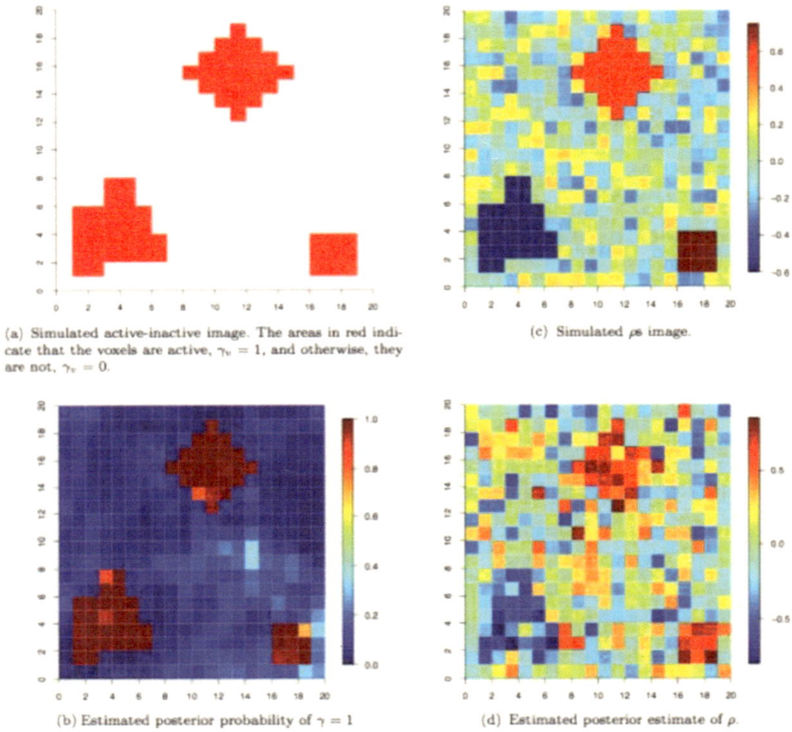

(a) Simulated active-inactive image. The areas in red indicate that the voxels are active, $\gamma_v = 1$, and otherwise, they are not, $\gamma_v = 0$.

(c) Simulated ρs image.

(b) Estimated posterior probability of $\gamma = 1$

(d) Estimated posterior estimate of ρ.

Figure 2. Simulated and estimated binary and ρ images.

4.3. Parcellation effect

In the previous simulations, image data was analysed together. In this simulation, we partition the data and then apply the proposed model to analyse each unit of the partitioned data. Our goal is to investigate the effect of the parcellation of an image on the estimation of active voxels. Given the binary image γ shown in **Figure 3(a)**, a unit of data is generated with the parameters being the same as the settings discussed in Section 3.1.

We consider four different parcellations, as shown in **Figure 3(a)**, **(b)** and **(d)**. **Table 2** shows the values of different measurements over 10 replications. Little difference can be found on the measures between different parcellations. However, the computational time is dramati-

http://dx.doi.org/10.5772/64823

cally reduced for case (d), where each parcellation contains fewer voxels. The same results in block and event-related fMRI experiments.

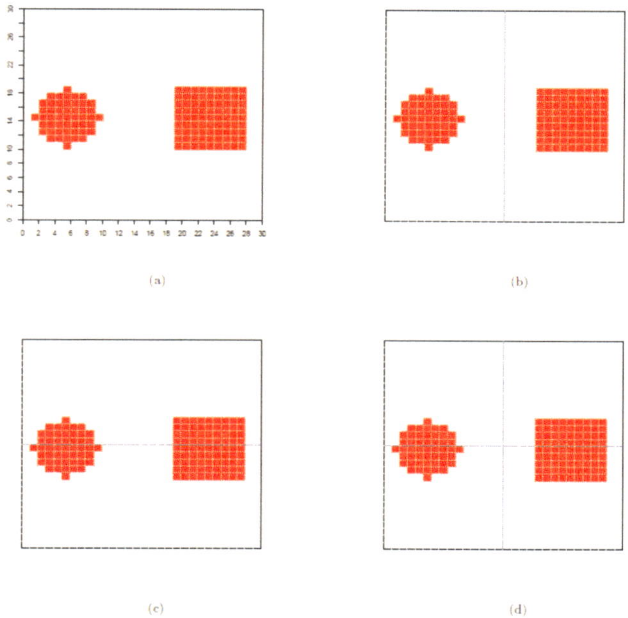

Figure 3. Four different parcellation schemes. The areas in red are active areas corresponding to $\gamma_v = 1$. The blue dashed line is used to partition the area into non-overlapping parts.

Parcellation Scheme	(a)	(b)	(c)	(d)
TCR	99.12 (98.61–99.84) %	99.07 (98.68–99.56) %	98.94 (98.03–99.64) %	99.08 (98.76–99.51) %
TPR	100%	100%	100%	100%
FPR	6.35 (1.51–9.97) %	6.68 (3.67–9.36) %	7.45 (3.12–13.87) %	5.82 (2.83–9.44) %
Running time ratio	8.75	2.75	2.75	1

The values within the parentheses are the ranges of different rates over 10 replications.

Table 2. The average percentage of correctly classified voxels (TCR), true positives (TPR), and false positives (FPR) over 10 replications for different image parcellations corresponding to **Figure 3(a)–(d)**.

4.4. A real-life simulation example

To further demonstrate the capability of the proposed model to accurately identify the activation regions, we simulate an fMRI dataset from an **R** package: **neuRosim** [28]. The simulated data follows the example of event-related fMRI study [24]. We consider four different tasks denoted by N1, N2, F1 and F2, which are presented randomly in the experiment. The onsets for each condition are schematically shown in **Figure 4**. We then specify three areas that are activated by the tasks shown in **Figure 5**. The simulated four-dimensional fMRI data consists of 351 scans, each containing three-dimensional image of size $53 \times 63 \times 46$ and being collected in every 2 s resulting the total time for the experiment is 11 min and 42 s.

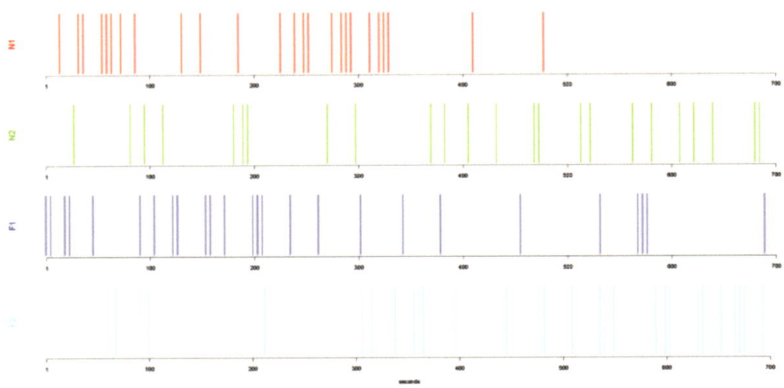

Figure 4. Depiction of temporal occurrences of four different tasks.

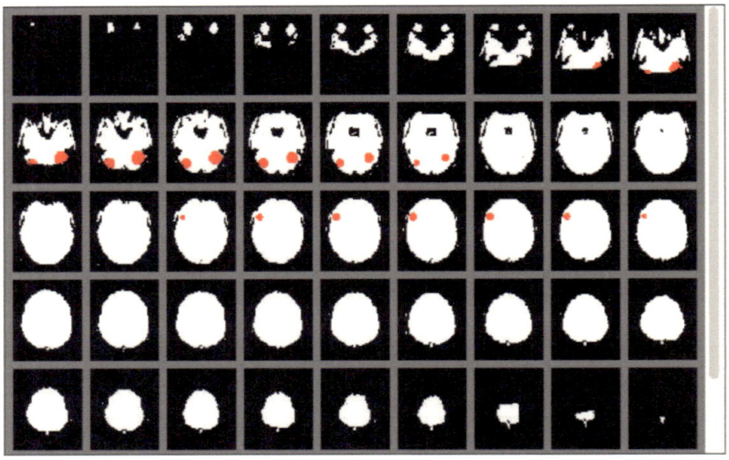

Figure 5. Activated regions upon representation of different tasks.

Now we apply the proposed model to analyse the simulated data. We split the array into disjointed arrays based on the Brodmann level regions. The voxel for all regions ranges from 236 to 969. We collect 1,000,000 samples to estimate the posterior probability of activation in each voxel. We consider the following probability:

$$P\left(\min_j \gamma_{vj} = 1 | y\right) \tag{19}$$

which is used to denote whether the voxel v is activated by any of applied stimuli. Once the posterior probability is greater than 0.8722, then the corresponding voxel is considered as activated by a stimulus. The activation maps registered into MNI 152 template (a reference brain map from the Montreal Neurological Institute) and the areas considered active are in yellow as shown in **Figure 6**. In addition to comparing specified activation regions in **Figure 5** to those detected in **Figure 6**, we also calculate the three measures, TCR, TPR and FPR which are 97.71%, 99.34% and 3.25%, respectively. The results show that proposed model performs well on classifying the active and inactive voxels.

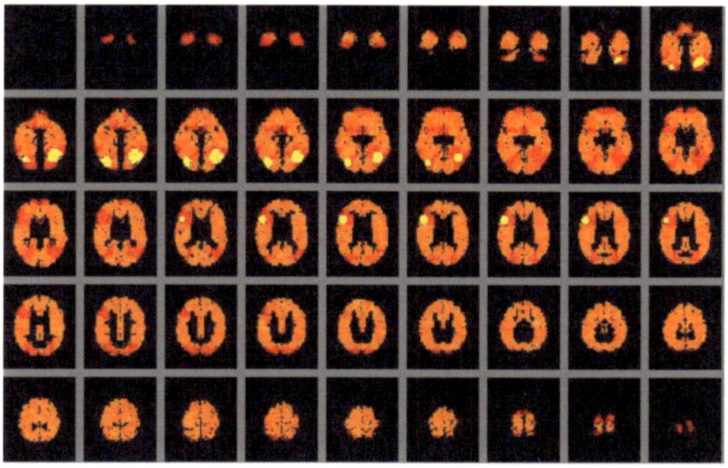

Figure 6. Estimated probability of activation in response to any face task with activation areas in yellow.

5. Application

We apply the spatial Bayesian variable selection approach discussed in Section 2 to real fMRI data, a study of the Simon effect [29]. In this Simon task, participants responded to one colour with the right hand, and to the other colour with the left hand. Congruence in this aspect means that a colour appears on the default side (congruent condition), or it may appear on the opposite side (incongruent condition). One participant's brain image data is selected to be analysed for the purpose of illustration. The four-dimensional fMRI BOLD image data was pre-processed using FSL from Oxford Centre for Functional MRI of the Brain [30], including motion correction, realignment, slice timing correction, spatial smoothing and high-pass filtering, before being analysed using our model. Incorrect trials were removed. The four tasks in this experiment were convolved with a double gamma function. We divided the pre-processed data into 48 Brodmann areas. The statistics of interest were registered into a standard template MNI152 for ease of visualization. We used a first-order temporal autocorrelation throughout the study.

We consider a voxel to be active when the posterior probability of γ_v is greater than c, which is either a deterministic value of 0.8722 [4] or is determined by an FDR equal to 0.05 [22]. However, in this event-related fMRI, 0.8722 seems too conservative, so the value of c is determined corresponding to an FDR equal to 0.05. The activation maps for different tasks are shown in **Figure 7(a)–(d)**.

One interesting question is to compare active domains corresponding to congruency. Posterior probabilities helped us find the following inequality between the incongruent and congruent tasks groups:

$$P\left(\beta_{\text{right-incon}} + \beta_{\text{left-incon}} > \beta_{\text{right-con}} + \beta_{\text{left-con}} | y\right), \tag{20}$$

where β_s is the magnitude of corresponding effect on the BOLD signal changes. The posterior activations are shown in **Figures 8** and **9** when posterior probabilities are thresholded by a critical value corresponding to FDR equal to 0.05. The active regions include frontal and occipital lobes detected by the models with and without consideration of spatial dependence of temporal correlations. These results are consistent with other studies [31, 32]. However, more active areas were detected by the model without consideration of spatial dependence of temporal correlations. For something like the Simon task, it is expected that the lateral prefrontal cortex to be activated as they are parts of the cognitive control network/multiple demand network, while the medial prefrontal cortex is part of the default mode network [33]. Therefore, it is possible that the activation in the medial part may be some spread of activity and therefore false positives. This is an important example that illustrates considering the

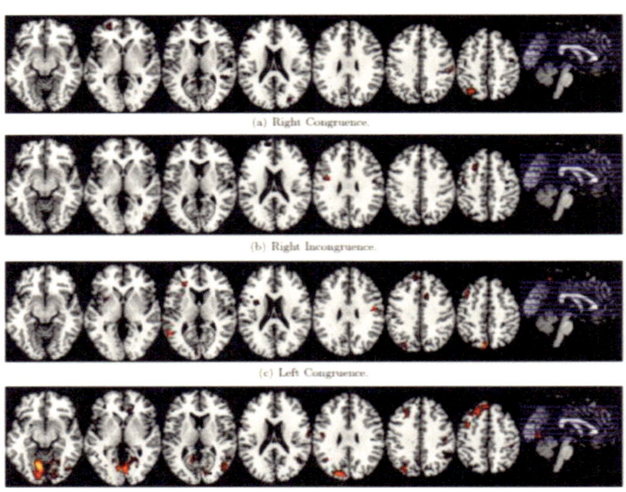

Figure 7. The activation areas with a posterior probability greater than c, corresponding to FDA = 0.05, shown in red for different tasks.

http://dx.doi.org/10.5772/64823

spatial dependence of temporal correlations may improve the estimation and reduce the some spurious detection of activation.

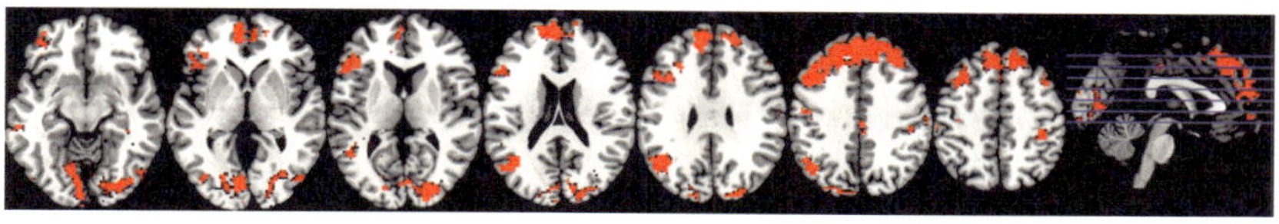

Figure 8. Areas shown more activity in incongruent than congruent task without consideration of spatial dependence of temporal correlations in the model.

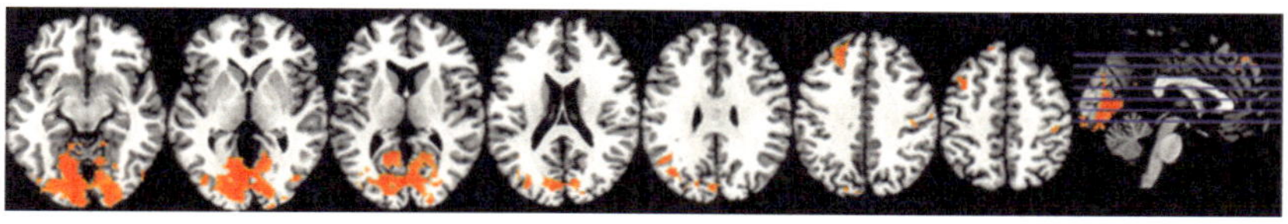

Figure 9. Areas shown more activity in incongruent than congruent task with consideration of spatial dependence of temporal correlations in the model.

6. Discussion and conclusions

In this work, we applied a new approach to performing Bayesian variable selection with consideration of spatial dependencies from both regression and temporal coefficients in single-subject event-related fMRI data. Through simulations, improvement in the detection of brain activity was observed for a wide range of different spatial structures, parcellations and experimental designs. We found that the proposed approach potentially decreases false positive rates as shown in **Table 1** in the simulation and **Figure 9** in the real example. In addition, prior information from brain structure and function for subject-level inference can be incorporated into the analysis.

It is worth noting that the proposed Bayesian approach partitions a brain into several regions before implementing the model to the fMRI data. In addition to Brodmann areas, several parcellations of the brain into distinct regions are available, such as the separate regions divided by a data-drive segmentation procedure using functional clustering. From the simulation study, we found the computational burden to be greatly reduced by the joint use of parcellation and an SGLMM. In particular, the probability of activation and activation magnitudes were readily computed without requiring an adjustment for multiple comparisons in a post-processing step. For broader goals, it would be of interest to extend the model to group studies. In addition, we are confident that Bayesian approaches represent an important direction in fMRI and in high-dimensional research in general.

Acknowledgements

This research was, in part, supported by the Ministry of Education, Taiwan, R.O.C. and National Cheng Kung University (the Aim for the Top University Project to National Cheng Kung University, NCKU). We thank the Mind Research and Imaging Center (MRIC) at NCKU for consultation and instrument availability.

Author details

Kuo-Jung Lee

Address all correspondence to: kuojunglee@mail.ncku.edu.tw

Department of Statistics, National Cheng-Kung University, Tainan, Taiwan

References

[1] J. A. Detre and T. Floyd. Functional MRI and its applications to the clinical neurosciences. The Neuroscientist. 2001;7:64–79.

[2] W. D. Penny, K. J. Friston, J. T. Ashburner, S. J. Kiebel, and T. E. Nichols, editors. Statistical Parametric Mapping: The Analysis of Functional Brain Images. London: Academic Press; 2006.

[3] K. J. Worsley, S. Marrett, P. Neelin, A. C. Vandal, K. J. Friston, and A. C. Evans. A unified statistical approach for determining significant voxels in images of cerebral activation. Human Brain Mapping. 1996;4:58–73.

[4] K. Lee, G. L. Jones, B. Caffo, and S. Bassett. Spatial Bayesian variable selection models on functional magnetic resonance imaging time-series data. Bayesian Analysis. 2014;9:699–732.

[5] L. Zhang, M. Guindani, and M. Vannucci. Bayesian models for functional magnetic resonance imaging data analysis. Wiley Interdisciplinary Reviews: Computational Statistics. 2015;7:21–41.

[6] M. Smith and L. Fahrmeir. Spatial Bayesian variable selection with application to functional magnetic resonance imaging. Journal of the American Statistical Association. 2007;102:417–431.

[7] J. Hughes and M. Haran. Dimension reduction and alleviation of confounding for spatial generalized linear mixed models. Journal of the Royal Statistical Society Series B. 2013;75:139–159.

[8] D. R. Musgrove, J. Hughes, and L. E. Eberly. Fast, fully Bayesian spatiotemporal inference for fMRI data. Biostatistics. 2016;17:291–303.

[9] M. Woolrich, M. Jenkinson, J. Brady, and S. Smith. Fully Bayesian spatio-temporal modeling for fMRI data. IEEE Transactions on Medical Imaging. 2004;23:213–231.

[10] A. Eklund, T. Nichols, M. Andersson, and H. Knutsson. Empirically investigating the statistical validity of SPM, FSL and AFNI for single subject fMRI analysis. In: 2015 IEEE 12th International Symposium on Biomedical Imaging (ISBI); New York, NY; 2015; pp. 1376–1380.

[11] A. Quirós, R. M. Diez, and D. Gamerman. Bayesian spatiotemporal model of fMRI data. NeuroImage. 2010;49:442–456.

[12] W.K. Hastings. Monte Carlo sampling methods using Markov chains and their applications. Biometrika. 1970;57:97–109.

[13] S. Brooks, A. Gelman, G. Jones, and X. Meng. Handbook of Markov Chain Monte Carlo. Chapman and Hall/CRC; 2011 Taylor & Francis Group, 6000 Broken Sound Parkway NW, Suite 300 Boca Raton, FL 33487–2742.

[14] W. D. Penny, N. J. Trujillo-Barreto, and K. J. Friston. Bayesian fMRI time series analysis with spatial priors. NeuroImage. 2005;24:350–362.

[15] M. A. Lindquist, J. M. Loh, L. Y. Atlas, and T. D. Wager. Modeling the hemodynamic response function in fMRI efficiency, bias and mis-modeling. NeuroImage. 2009;45:S187–S198.

[16] J. C. Rajapakse, F. Kruggel, and J. M. M. D. Y. Cramon. Modeling hemodynamic response for analysis of functional MRI time-series. Human Brain Mapping. 1998;6:283–300.

[17] E. I. George and R. E. McCulloch. Approaches for Bayesian variable selection. Statistica Sinica. 1997;7:339–374.

[18] D. M. Cvetkovć, M. Doob, and H. Sachs. Spectra of Graphs: Theory and Applications. 3rd ed. New York, NY: Wiley; 1998.

[19] N. G. Best, L. Waller, A. Thomas, E. M. Conlon, and R. Arnold. Discussion of Bayesian models for spatially correlated disease and exposure data. In: J. O. Berger, A. P. Dawid, and A. F. M. Smith, editors. Bayesian Statistics 6. Oxford University Press; 1999. pp. 147–150.

[20] A. Shmuel, E. Yacoub, D. Chaimow, N. K. Logothetis, and K. Ugurbil. Spatio-temporal point-spread function of fMRI signal in human gray matter at 7 Tesla. NeuroImage. Oxford 2007;35:539–552.

[21] M. Barbieri and J. O. Berger. Optimal predictive model selection. Annals of Statistics. 2004;32:870–897.

[22] S. Kalus, P. G. Sämann, and L. Fahrmeir. Classification of brain activation via spatial Bayesian variable selection in fMRI regression. Advances in Data Analysis and Classification. 2014;8:63–83.

[23] Y. Benjamini and Y. Hochberg. Controlling the false discovery rate: a practical and powerful approach to multiple testing. Journal of the Royal Statistical Society, Series B. 1995;57:289–300.

[24] R. Henson, T. Shallice, M. Gorno-Tempini, and R. Dolan. Face repetition effects in implicit and explicit memory tests as measured by fMRI. Cerebral Cortex. 2002;12:178–186.

[25] G. Jones, M. Haran, B. Caffo, and R. Neath. Fixed-width output analysis for Markov chain Monte Carlo. Journal of the American Statistical Association. 2006;101:1537–1547.

[26] O. Josephs and R. Henson. Event-related fMRI: modelling, inference and optimisation. The Royal Society: Philosophical Transactions B. 1999;354:1215–1228.

[27] M. Bezener, J. Hughes, and G. L. Jones. Bayesian spatiotemporal modeling using hierarchical spatial priors with applications to functional magnetic resonance imaging. Available from: http://users.stat.umn.edu/~galin/.

[28] M. Welvaert, J. Durnez, B. Moerkerke, G. Berdoolaege, and Y. Rosseel. neuRosim: An R package for generating fMRI data. Journal of Statistical Software. 2011;44:1–18.

[29] T. Wen and S. Hsieh. Neuroimaging of the joint Simon effect with believed biological and non-biological co-actors. Frontiers in Human Neuroscience. 2015;9:1–13.

[30] FMRIB, Oxford, UK. FMRIB Software Library [Internet]. Available from: http://fsl.fmrib.ox.ac.uk/fsl/fslwiki/.

[31] X. Liu, M. Banich, M. Jacobson, and J. Tanabe. Common and distinct neural substrates of attentional control in an integrated Simon and spatial Stroop task as assessed by event-related fMRI. NeuroImage. 2004;22:1097–1106.

[32] B.U. Forstmann, W. P. M van den Wildenberg, and K. R. Riderinkhof. Neural mechanisms, temporal dynamics, and individual differences in interference control. Neuroscience. 2008;20:1854–1865.

[33] T. A. Niendam, A. R. Laird, K. L. Ray, Y. M. Dean, D. C. Glahn, and C. S. Carter. Meta-analytic evidence for a superordinate cognitive control network subserving diverse executive functions. Cognitive, Affective, and Behavioural Neuroscience. 2012;12:241–268.

[34] A. Gelman, J. C. Carlin, H. Stern, D. Dunson, A. Vehtari, and D. Rubin. Bayesian Data Analysis. 3rd ed. Chapman and Hall/CRC; 2013.

[35] C. Berrett and C. A. Calder. Bayesian spatial binary classification. Spatial Statistics. 2016;16:72–102.

Chapter 5

Texture Analysis in Magnetic Resonance Imaging: Review and Considerations for Future Applications

Andrés Larroza, Vicente Bodí and David Moratal

Additional information is available at the end of the chapter

http://dx.doi.org/10.5772/64641

Abstract

Texture analysis is a technique used for the quantification of image texture. It has been successfully used in many fields, and in the past years it has been applied in magnetic resonance imaging (MRI) as a computer-aided diagnostic tool. Quantification of the intrinsic heterogeneity of different tissues and lesions is necessary as they are usually imperceptible to the human eye. In the present chapter, we describe texture analysis as a process consisting of six steps: MRI acquisition, region of interest (ROI) definition, ROI preprocessing, feature extraction, feature selection, and classification. There is a great variety of methods and techniques to be chosen at each step and all of them can somehow affect the outcome of the texture analysis application. We reviewed the literature regarding texture analysis in clinical MRI focusing on the important considerations to be taken at each step of the process in order to obtain maximum benefits and to avoid misleading results.

Keywords: texture analysis, magnetic resonance imaging, classification, computer aided diagnosis, segmentation

1. Introduction

Magnetic resonance imaging (MRI) has become a powerful diagnostic tool by providing high quality images, thanks to new advances in technology. MRI offers excellent anatomic details due to its high soft-tissue contrast and the possibility to enhance different types of tissues using different acquisition protocols. However, diagnosis of some pathologies remains difficult due to the restricted ability of the human eye to detect intrinsic, heterogeneous characteristics of certain tissues. For example, the visual appearance on MRI of a metastatic brain tumor can be very similar to one of a radionecrosis lesion (**Figure 1**), and a wrong diagnosis can lead to improper patient treatment. In these particular cases, histopathology remains the gold standard diagnostic technique. In an effort to avoid this invasive diagnostic approach, and considering that additional imaging modalities are costly and not as widely available as conventional MRI, great interest exists in identifying reliable imaging features from routine MRI scans that would help differentiate certain lesions [1].

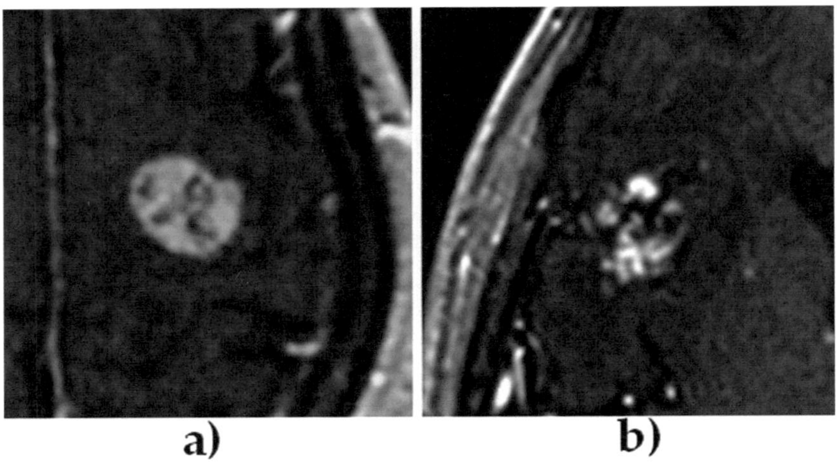

Figure 1. T1-weighted MRI with contrast enhancement of a brain metastatic lesion (a), and a radionecrosis lesion (b). Discrimination of these different entities is crucial for patient treatment but it is visually non-feasible. Texture analysis has demonstrated to be a useful tool for this purpose [1, 19].

Computer-aided diagnostic tools assist the radiologist in the diagnosis by providing quantitative measures of morphology, function, and other biomarkers in different tissues. In the past years, texture analysis has gained attention in medical applications and has been proved to be a significant computer-aided diagnostic tool [2]. There is not a strict definition of an image texture but it can be described as the spatial arrangement of patterns that provides the visual appearance of coarseness, randomness, smoothness, etc. [3]. Texture analysis describes a wide range of techniques for quantification of gray-level patterns and pixel inter-relationships within an image providing a measure of heterogeneity. It has been shown that different image areas exhibit different textural patterns that are sometimes imperceptible to the human eye [2].

Applications of texture analysis in medical imaging include classification and segmentation of tissues and lesions. A search of papers containing the keywords "texture" and "MRI" in the title was performed in SciVerse Scopus[1] retrieving 200 papers on January 19th 2016, of which 140 were original studies dealing with texture analysis in clinical MRI. The distribution of these studies per organ is shown in **Figure 2**. It is clear that there is an increased interest in texture analysis in recent years, and that the major attention has been paid to neurological applications. Some brain applications include discrimination between different types of tumors [4, 5],

[1] https://www.scopus.com

classification of diseases like Alzheimer's [6] or Friedreich ataxia [7], and brain segmentation [8, 9]. Following brain studies, we found applications in liver, breast, and prostate [10–12], and cardiac MRI for detection of scarred myocardium and classification of patients with low and high risk of arrhythmias [13, 14].

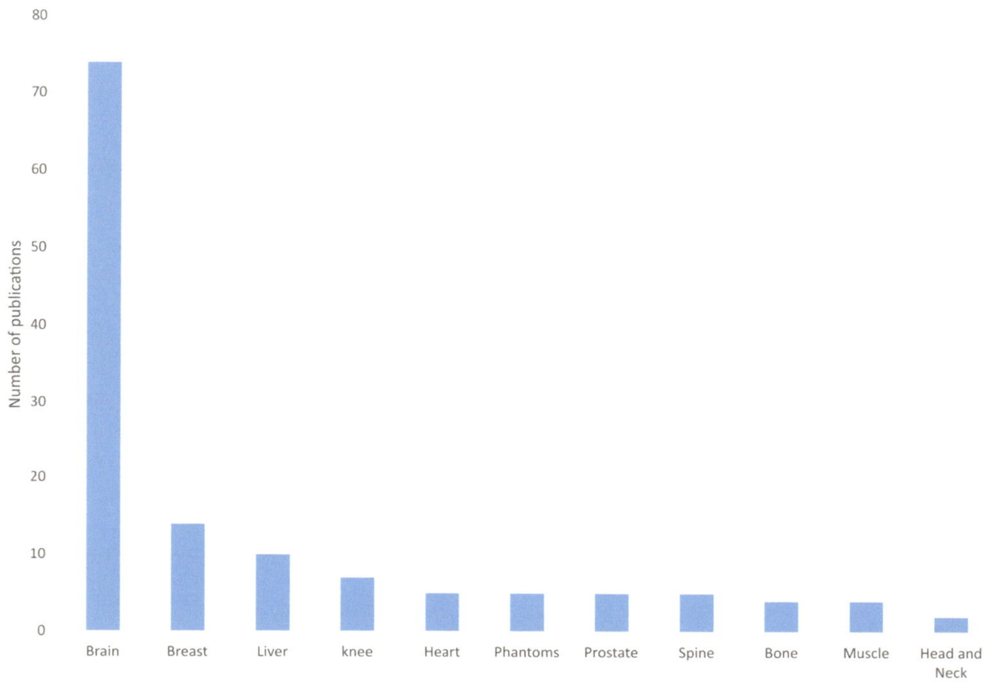

Figure 2. Distribution of original publications regarding texture analysis in MRI according to the studied organ.

This work is presented as a literature review of the most relevant publications regarding texture analysis in MRI. Rather than providing a detailed summary of the state of the art found in the literature search, we focused this work on the process of texture analysis considering papers that compared different methods so we can have an idea of the best approaches for certain applications.

2. Texture analysis process

Texture analysis applications involve a process that consists of six steps: MRI acquisition, region of interest (ROI) definition, ROI preprocessing, feature extraction, feature selection, and classification (**Figure 3**). None of these steps is specific, and the methods have to be chosen according to the application. The texture outcome can be considerably affected depending on the methodology used throughout the process. Herein, we present a condensed description of each step of the texture analysis process focusing on applications that compared different scenarios or methods.

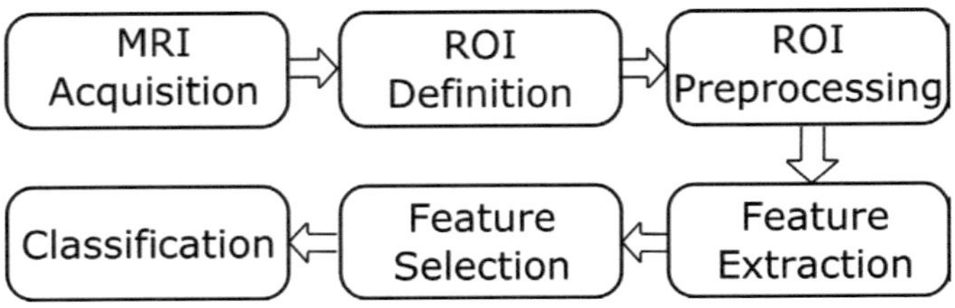

Figure 3. Main steps for MRI classification by means of texture analysis. ROI: region of interest.

2.1. MRI acquisition

Magnetic resonance imaging is widely used nowadays because of its high soft-tissue contrast and the possibility to enhance specific tissues by varying the acquisition sequence parameters. In this respect, the outcome of texture analysis strongly relies on the image acquisition protocols, and these should be carefully selected in order to obtain maximum accuracy and reproducibility. Different measuring techniques produce different patterns in texture and these may vary among centers and manufacturers [15]. Texture analysis can be used reliably at one center with a specific imaging protocol but this does not mean that the same methodology can be directly applied to images acquired at different centers with different protocols [16].

2.1.1. Sequences

Three relevant MRI tissue parameters can be measured in a typical spin echo (SE) sequence: spin density (ρ), spin-lattice relaxation time (T1), and spin-spin relaxation time (T2); each of them showing different image contrast and texture. Examples of MR images weighted in these three parameters are shown in **Figure 4**. Other imaging techniques, like the gradient echo (GE) fast low angle shot (FLASH), introduce significant effects on image texture due to their own measuring characteristics [17]. Repetition time (TR), bandwidth/echo time (BW/TE), and flip angle are the properties that are most likely altered in a clinical setting. Repetition time had the biggest impact when comparing different foam phantoms using clinical breast MRI protocols, whereby better texture discrimination was elicited at higher TR [18].

The choice of the MRI sequence for texture analysis depends on the application. Contrast-enhanced T1-weighted images is the current standard MRI protocol used by clinicians to assess brain tumors and was used for texture analysis in [1, 4]. Some studies compared different modalities obtaining diverse results. In the study of Tiwari et al. [19], contrast-enhanced T1-weighted images provided better performance over T2-weighted and fluid-attenuated inversion recovery (FLAIR) images for discrimination of recurrent brain tumors from radiation-induced lesions. T1-weighted MRI was also notably better than FLAIR images for dementia classification [20]. T2-weigthed images were more suitable for differentiation between benign and malignant tumors [21, 22], and for discrimination of posterior fossa tumors in children [23]. Texture analysis applied to diffusion-weighted images also proved to be efficient for brain tumor classification [24–26]. Texture features used in these studies differ from each other, so a definite assumption of which MRI sequence is better cannot be made.

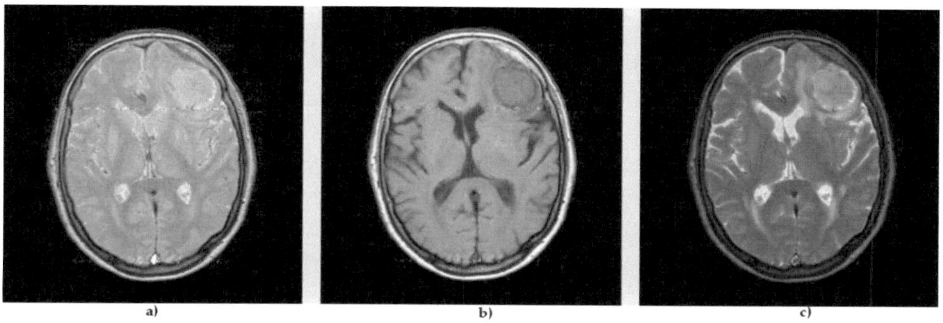

Figure 4. Spin echo images of a patient with meningioma. (a), ρ-image (TR/TE = 2000 ms/10 ms). (b), T1 image (TR/TE = 600 ms/10 ms). (c), T2 image (TR/TE 2000 ms/100 ms). TR: repetition time, TE: spin echo time. Reproduced with the permission of the publisher (Les Laboratories Servier ©, Suresnes, France) from [17].

2.1.2. Influence of spatial resolution and signal-to-noise ratio

Spatial resolution and signal-to-noise ratio (SNR) have been reported to be the most influential factors for texture analysis [15, 27, 28]. Image resolution is defined by slice thickness, field of view (FOV), and matrix size. Signal-to-noise ratio is defined as the coefficient between the mean signal over a homogeneous region of a tissue of interest and the standard deviation of the background noise. Texture discrimination improves with higher levels of SNR and it has been reported that a SNR > 4 is necessary to measure the real textural behavior of the human brain [17]. Discrimination based on texture analysis also improves with higher spatial resolution, as shown by Jirak et al. [29], who found the best separation of three different phantoms at a pixel resolution of 0.45×0.45 mm^2 (good separation was also found at 0.77×0.90 mm^2, whereas the worst discrimination was for the lowest tested resolution of 1.53×1.80 mm^2). Texture analysis fails if the image resolution is insufficient since the finest textural details cannot be spotted. Texture features from higher spatial resolution images are more sensitive to variations in the acquisition parameters. In [28], it was found that the least influenced resolution was at 0.8×0.8 mm^2.

Although current routine MRI scanners can produce high-resolution images, these are susceptible to motion artifacts, given the long scan times and are not widespread in clinical practice. In [30], they found a strong correlation between 3D structural indices and 3D texture features in trabecular bone in osteoporosis using routine, low-resolution images (0.7 mm), indicating that these can be used to quantify the bone architecture without the need of higher resolution images. These previous results indicate that even if high-resolution images provide better texture discrimination, its application in clinical practice is far complicated as no good reproducibility among centers is expected. Apparently the slice thickness does not influence significantly the outcome of 2D texture analysis according to Savio et al. [31], who found only moderate differences between 1 mm and 3 mm thickness for separation of white matter tissue and multiple sclerosis plaques.

2.1.3. Influence of field strength

One important difference among MRI scanners is the field strength of the magnet, the most common values in clinical routine nowadays being those of 1.5T and 3T. Scanners with higher field strength provide more SNR, thus increasing spatial and temporal resolution. In counterpart, artifacts resulting from breathing or any other type of body motion are more prominent on 3T than on 1.5T scanners, but these are generally compensated using some techniques offered by manufacturers [32]. Better texture-based discrimination is expected on the higher quality images acquired on 3T scanners as it was reported for liver fibrosis [33] and breast cancer classification [34]. In [22], they found significant differences between 1.5T and 3T when squamous cell carcinoma tumors on head and neck were compared. However, their results are in contrast with previous evidence [33, 34] since benign versus malignant tumor discrimination was better on 1.5T. In the study performed by Waugh et al. [18], texture discrimination of foam phantoms using different clinical breast MRI protocols was in general improved when a 3T scanner was used, but changes in the imaging parameters at 1.5T had less influence on the texture outcome.

2.1.4. Multicenter studies

Few multicenter studies regarding the application of texture analysis in MRI have been published. In [21], they concluded that texture analysis on MRI can discriminate between different brain tissues obtained in routine procedures at three different centers. In [16], they compared the classification performance to discriminate between bone marrow and fat tissue on T1-weighted MRI of knees from 63 patients obtained from three centers with two different field strength MRI scanners: two centers at 1T and one at 3T. Texture information was extracted from two centers and was used to predict tissue using data from the third center, concluding that feature sets from one center may be used for tissue discrimination in data from other centers. Pixel size was found to be the parameter that mostly influences the texture outcome. In a very large multicenter study, Karimaghaloo et al. [8] analyzed 2380 scans from 247 different centers for segmentation of multiple sclerosis lesions achieving an overall sensitivity of 95% on a separate dataset of 120 scans from 24 centers. The promising results of this study may be the consequence of extracting texture features from different MRI protocols (T1, T2, proton density, and FLAIR) and using them in combination when modeling the classifier. It should also be noted that images were corrected for nonuniformity effects and were normalized into a common spatial and intensity space, thus reducing the possible differences among multicenter scans. Opposite conclusions were reached by Fruehwald-Pallamar et al. [22], as they stated that texture analysis is useful for discrimination of benign and malignant tumors when using one scanner with the same protocol, but it is not recommended for multicenter studies. However, they did not mention any image normalization or inhomogeneity correction that could somehow have affected their results, as we discuss in Section 2.3.

2.2. Region of interest definition

Texture features are computed inside a predefined region of interest (ROI), or volume or interest (VOI) in the case of 3D texture analysis, and are usually placed over a homogeneous tissue or lesion area. Manual definition of ROIs is still considered the gold standard in many applications, and it is the chosen option over automatic methods [35–38]. Different approaches have been used to define ROIs that are also extended to 3D texture analysis. One approach for ROI definition is the positioning of squares [39] or circles [40] of predefined sizes over the tissue to be analyzed. Using this approach, only information of the underlying tissue is captured but some texture details can be lost because the ROI does not cover the entire area of interest. Another alternative is to use a bounding box defined as the smallest enclosing rectangular area of the tissue of interest [41, 42]. The latter approach has the advantage that it covers the entire tissue or lesion, however it also includes information from adjacent parts that can affect texture quantification. Although delineation of the entire tissue or lesion can be tedious, it is a better approach since the whole area of interest is included [23, 43]. In [44], they studied the effect of lesion segmentation on the diagnostic accuracy to discriminate benign and malignant breast lesions. They concluded that for both 2D and 3D texture analysis, delineation of the entire lesion provides better accuracy than the bounding box approach. **Figure 5** shows examples of the three aforementioned ROI definition approaches.

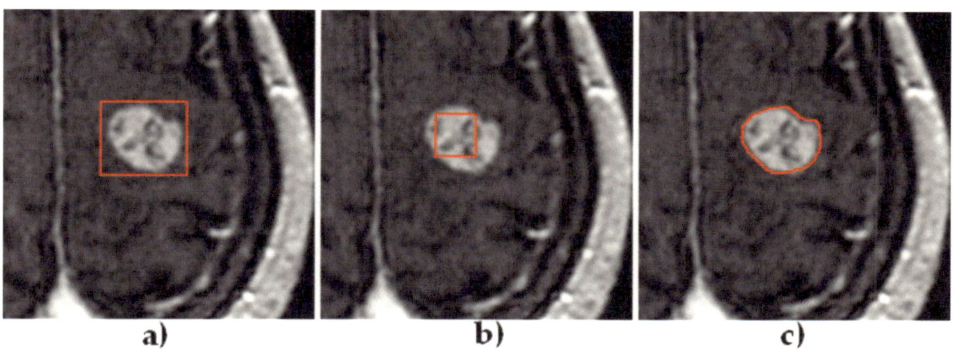

Figure 5. Approaches for defining a region of interest (ROI) over a brain tumor. The use of a bounding box that covers the entire lesion (a), or a small square inside the tumor (b) can be defined quickly and easily, but the delineation of the entire lesion (c) is preferred in order to capture the maximum texture information only within the area of interest.

2.2.1. Size of the region of interest

The size of the ROI should be sufficiently large to capture the texture information thereby eliciting statistical significance [45]. In [46], they studied the effect of ROI size on various texture features extracted from circular ROIs of 10 different sizes on brain MRI of healthy adults. They concluded that the effect of size becomes insignificant when large ROIs are used. In general, texture features were highly affected at ROI areas smaller than 80 × 80 pixels and became unaffected at ROI areas of around 180 × 180 pixels. These results are in general true for certain texture features but they can vary among the extensive range of available texture analysis methods. In Section 2.4 we discuss the texture analysis methods mostly applied in MRI. It is also important to notice that the ROI size might depend on the MRI acquisition parameters. It is not the same to use a ROI of 180 × 180 pixels area over an image region of 1.5 × 1.5 mm^2 resolution than over an image of 0.5 × 0.5 mm^2. The MR images used by Sikiö et al. [46] had a pixel size of 0.5 × 0.7 mm^2 with a slice thickness of 4.0 mm. A good methodology to avoid possible influences of ROI size might be the use of squares and circles of the same size among all the studied samples but as we mentioned before, complete delineation of the ROI might offer better results. We recommend the use of the ROI delineation approach when the range of lesion sizes among samples is not significantly broad and when the employed texture features are not affected between this range, otherwise ROIs of the same size might be a better approach.

2.2.2. Feature maps

Texture feature maps can be computed by defining ROIs as sliding blocks of $n \times n$ pixels centered at each pixel on the image, so for each pixel a specific texture feature value is computed including its surrounding neighborhood. The block size should be large enough to capture sufficient texture information from each pixel neighborhood, but small enough to capture more local characteristics allowing finer detection of regions [45]. **Figure 6** shows examples of texture maps computed for sliding blocks of different sizes. Texture maps can reveal some characteristics that are not visible on the original image and are mainly used for segmentation tasks [47]. Computing features over texture maps can lead to better results than using the original MR images [48].

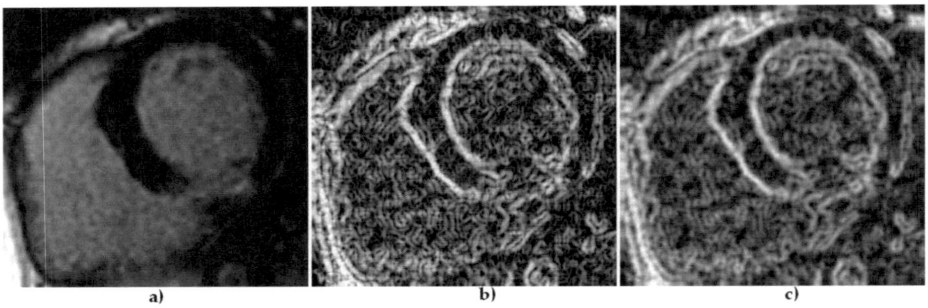

Figure 6. Texture feature maps of a cardiac MR image: (a) original image, (b) entropy feature map computed with a sliding block with a size of 5 × 5 pixels, and (c) entropy feature map computed with a sliding block of 9 × 9 pixels.

2.3. Region of interest preprocessing

It is clear from Section 2.1 that MRI acquisition protocols are relevant for texture analysis. Several preprocessing techniques have been proposed in order to minimize the effects of acquisition protocols and are especially important when dealing with multicenter studies. The main purpose of these preprocessing techniques is to put all ROIs in the same condition, so features extracted from them represent essentially the texture being examined. Some preprocessing methods also aim to improve the texture discrimination. For example, Assefa et al. [49] extracted texture features from a power map computed from the localized Hartley transform of the image, and Chen et al. [50] computed features from ROIs defined over texture maps.

2.3.1. Interpolation

Image spatial resolution is one of the most influential factors in texture analysis, and it was demonstrated that higher resolutions tend to improve texture-based classification, but high-resolution images are not usually available in clinical routine [29, 30]. Image interpolation is an option to enhance images with a low spatial resolution. The effect of image interpolation on texture features was analyzed by Mayerhoefer et al. [51] comparing three interpolation methods applied on T2-weighted images acquired at five different resolutions. They concluded that MR image interpolation has the potential to improve the results of texture-based classification, recommending a maximum interpolation factor of four. In their study, the most considerable improvements were found when images with an original resolution of 0.94×0.94 mm^2 and 0.47×0.47 mm^2, respectively, were interpolated by factors of two or four using the zero-fill interpolation technique at the *k-space* level. Image interpolation is of special interest when dealing with 3D texture analysis because in most MRI sequences the slice thickness is larger than the in-plane resolution. Re-slicing all images to obtain isotropic image resolution is required for computing textures feature to ensure the conservation of scales and directions in all three dimensions [52].

2.3.2. Normalization

It was demonstrated that some features are not only dependent on texture, but also on other ROI properties, such as the mean intensity and variance [53]. To avoid the influence of such factors, ROI normalization is a recommended preprocessing step (**Figure 7**). In [54], they studied the effects of ROI normalization on texture classification of T2-weighted images and demonstrated that classification errors were dependent on the MR acquisition protocols if no normalization was applied. They compared three methods, and the one that yielded the best results is known as the "$\pm 3\sigma$" normalization. In this method, image intensities are normalized between $\mu \pm 3\sigma$, where μ is the mean value of gray-levels inside the ROI, and σ is the standard deviation, so that gray-levels located outside the range $[\mu - 3\sigma, \mu + 3\sigma]$ are not considered for further analysis. Enhancement of the variations in gray-levels between neighbors is a favorable factor for improving the classification performance. The "$\pm 3\sigma$" normalization technique has become the most popular and preferred choice in most publications [1, 55–57]. In another study, Loizou et al. [58] compared six MRI normalization methods applied to T2-weighted MR images from patients with multiple sclerosis and healthy volunteers. They concluded that a method based on normalization of the whole brain, in which the original histogram is stretched and shifted in order to cover a wider dynamic range, is the most appropriate for the assessment of multiple sclerosis brain lesions by means of texture analysis.

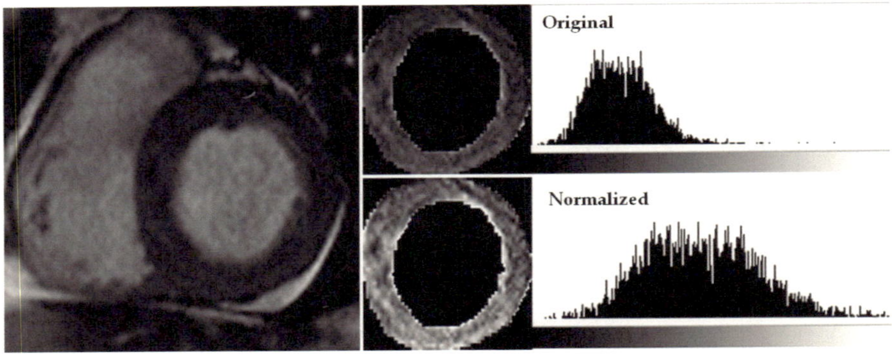

Figure 7. Example of region of interest (ROI) normalization of a cardiac MR image. The extracted ROI is shown in the original histogram and after normalization using the "±3σ" method.

2.3.3. Inhomogeneity correction

There is still another residual effect that is not eliminated by ROI normalization, which is the variation of intensity present in MR images mainly caused by static magnetic field inhomogeneity and imperfections of the radiofrequency coils [17]. **Figure 8** shows examples of liver MRI affected by nonuniformity artifacts. Texture features depend on local average image intensity and are therefore affected by image inhomogeneity. Correction of nonuniformity artifacts in MRI is recommended as a preprocessing step prior to ROI normalization and especially for large ROIs [59]. A review of methods for MRI inhomogeneity correction is available in [60], the most popular method found in texture literature [61–64] being the so-called N3 algorithm [65].

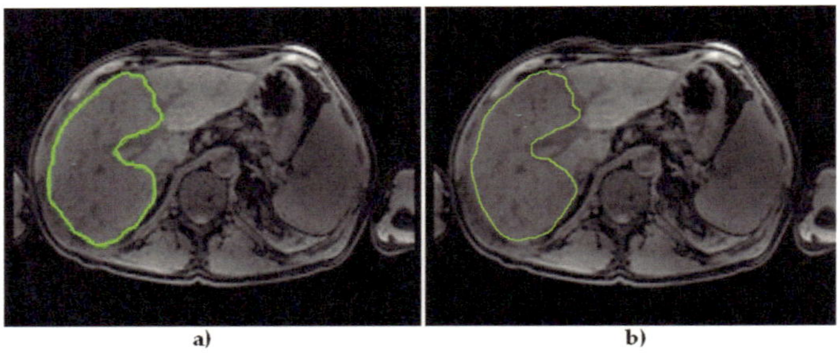

Figure 8. Example of a liver MRI with inhomogeneity (a), the average local image intensity of the lower left part is darker than the upper part. The corrected image is shown in (b). Reproduced with permission from [59].

2.3.4. Quantization of gray-levels

Texture analysis methods based on matrix computation, e.g., co-occurrence and run-length matrices, require the quantization of gray-levels. A typical MR image is represented by 10 or 12 bits per pixel, that is, 1024 or 4096 levels of gray. So, in MRI texture analysis, quantization will refer to the reduction of levels of gray used to represent the image. Typical numbers of gray-levels used for texture feature computation are 16, 32, 64, 128, and 256. Reducing the number of gray-levels improves SNR and the counting statistics inherent in the matrix-based texture analysis method at the expense of discriminatory power [66]. Some studies reported that no significant effects were found when a different number of gray levels were tested [55, 67] while in the study of Chen et al. [44], a gray-level number of 32 was reported to be an optimal choice for breast MRI. A specific study regarding the impact of the number of gray-levels on co-occurrence matrix texture features was carried out by Mahmoud-Ghoneim et al. [68]. They concluded that the number of gray levels, or dynamic range, has a significant influence on the classification of brain white matter, obtaining an optimal number of 128 levels for both 2D and 3D texture analysis approaches. It is recommended to optimize the number of gray levels for each specific application.

2.4. Feature extraction

Feature extraction is the main and specific step in the texture analysis process and implies the computation of texture features from predefined ROIs. Many approaches have been proposed in order to quantify the texture of an image allowing the computation of numerous features. In this section, we briefly describe the most popular texture analysis methods that were successfully used to characterize MRI tissues. A review of existing feature extraction methods can be found in [69, 70]. Although methods based on the first order statistics (histogram features) are normally used in combination with other methods, as they may improve the texture-based classification or segmentation [10, 71–73], they are not presented here as they do not really describe the actual texture of the image or ROI being analyzed [70].

2.4.1. Statistical methods

Statistical methods represent the texture by considering the distributions and relationships between the gray-levels of an image. Hereby we briefly describe a method based on second-order statistics, the co-occurrence matrix, a method based on higher-order statistics, namely the run-length matrix, and a method that combines the statistical approach with the structural properties of the image known as local binary patterns (LBP).

2.4.1.1. Co-occurrence matrix

The co-occurrence matrix allows extraction of statistical information regarding the distribution of pixel pairs in the image. Pairs of pixels separated by a predefined distance and direction are counted and the resulting values are allocated in the co-occurrence matrix. The count is based on the number of pairs of pixels that have the same distribution of gray-level values [3]. Normally, co-occurrence matrices are computed in four directions (horizontal, vertical, 45°, 135°) for 2D, and in 13 directions for 3D approaches [52], using different pixel or voxel separations. Features originally proposed by Haralick *et al.* [74, 75] are then computed for each co-occurrence matrix. **Figure 9** shows an example of computation of the co-occurrence matrix.

The pixel distance has to be chosen according to the application: a larger distance will allow detection of coarse areas but care must be taken not to overstep the size of the ROIs.

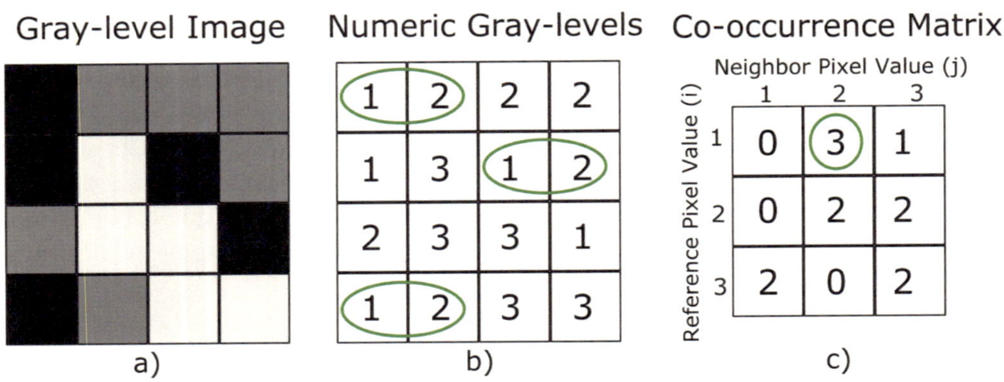

Figure 9. Computation of a co-occurrence matrix for a given 4 × 4 pixel image (a) with three gray-levels (b). In this example, the matrix is computed in horizontal direction for one pixel separation. The number of transitions of gray-levels is counted and allocated in the co-occurrence matrix (c). The circled values indicate that there are three transitions from one to two gray levels and this count is allocated in the corresponding position in the co-occurrence matrix.

One main concern about matrix-based texture features is their dependence on direction, so different values may be obtained if the image is rotated. This is unacceptable for texture characterization on MRI since images from different patients may have different orientations. Rotation-invariant features can be achieved by averaging each matrix value over all directions [44, 49] or by averaging the statistical features derived from the co-occurrence matrices [47]. Texture features based on co-occurrence matrices have become the most popular method and have been proven to be useful for classification of tissues and lesions in MRI [76–81].

2.4.1.2. Run-length matrix

Run-length matrices consider higher-order statistical information in comparison with co-occurrence matrices. Runs of a specific gray-level are counted for a chosen direction. For example, three consecutive pixels with the same gray-level value along the horizontal direction constitutes one run of length three. Computation of a simple run-length matrix is shown in **Figure 10**. Fine textures will be dominated by short runs whereas coarse textures will include longer runs [69]. The features originally proposed by Galloway [82] are usually computed for ROI characterization. Rotation invariance can be achieved by averaging over all directions, as previously mentioned for the co-occurrence matrix method.

There is one important consideration about run-length matrix features. As demonstrated by Sikiö et al. [46], the features run-length nonuniformity (RLN) and gray-level nonuniformity (GLN) were linearly dependent on the ROI size. The linear behavior of these nonuniform features is due to the original mathematical definition, which squares the number of gray-levels (N_g) for each run length (Eq. (1)) or the number of run-lengths (N_r) for each gray-level (Eq. (2)). Thus, for a larger ROI there will be more runs. The normalization factor C (Eq. (3)) is correlated with the number of pixels and not its square. Using the square of the normalization factor C, as proposed by Loh et al. [83], is a recommended approach in order to reduce the dependence on ROI size.

$$RLN = C^{-1}\sum_{j=1}^{N_r}\left[\sum_{i=1}^{N_g} p(i,j)\right]^2 \tag{1}$$

$$GLN = C^{-1}\sum_{i=1}^{N_g}\left[\sum_{j=1}^{N_r} p(i,j)\right]^2 \tag{2}$$

$$C = \sum_{i=1}^{N_g}\sum_{j=1}^{N_r} p(i,j) \tag{3}$$

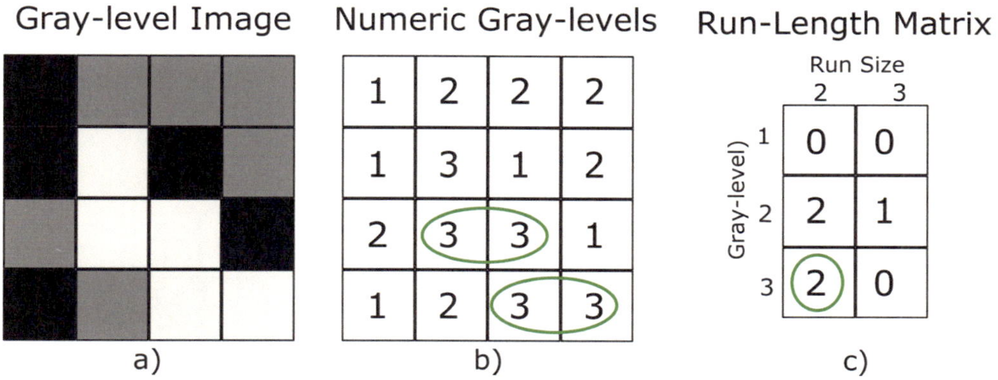

Figure 10. Computation of a run-length matrix for a given 4 × 4 pixels image (a) with three different gray-levels (b). The number of runs for each gray-level is allocated in the run-length matrix (c). For example, there are two runs of size two for the gray-level of three (circled values).

2.4.1.3. Local binary patterns

The local binary pattern (LBP) is a texture descriptor introduced by Ojala et al. [84] and it became very popular, thanks to its simplicity and high-discriminative power. The LBP descriptor labels each pixel in an image by comparing its gray-level with the surrounding pixels and then assigning a binary number. A value of unity is assigned to the surrounding neighbors with gray-level greater than the central pixel in a predefined patch and a value of zero otherwise. A binary number is then obtained and assigned to the central pixel. The original LBP operator considers a 3 × 3 patch, so the surrounding pixels form a binary number of 8 digits. After labeling all pixels in an image, a LBP feature map is obtained as well as a histogram that consists of 256 bins when considering 3 × 3 patch. **Figure 11** summarizes the described steps. The LBP histogram can be used as feature vector for classification where each bin represents one feature. Another approach is to compute new features from the LBP map as carried out by Oppedal et al. [20] and Sheethal et al. [85]. Uniform LBPs have been proposed to reduce the length of the feature histogram. A LBP binary code is uniform if it contains at most two transitions from 0 to 1 or vice-versa. Examples of uniform patterns are: 0000000 (no transitions), 00001111 (one transition), and 10001111 (two transitions). Patterns with more than two transitions are labeled as nonuniform, and distinct labels are assigned to each uniform pattern. For a 3 × 3 patch, the number of bins on the uniform histogram is reduced to 59 instead of the original 256. Uniform LBP patterns function as templates for microstructures, such as spots, edges, corners, etc.

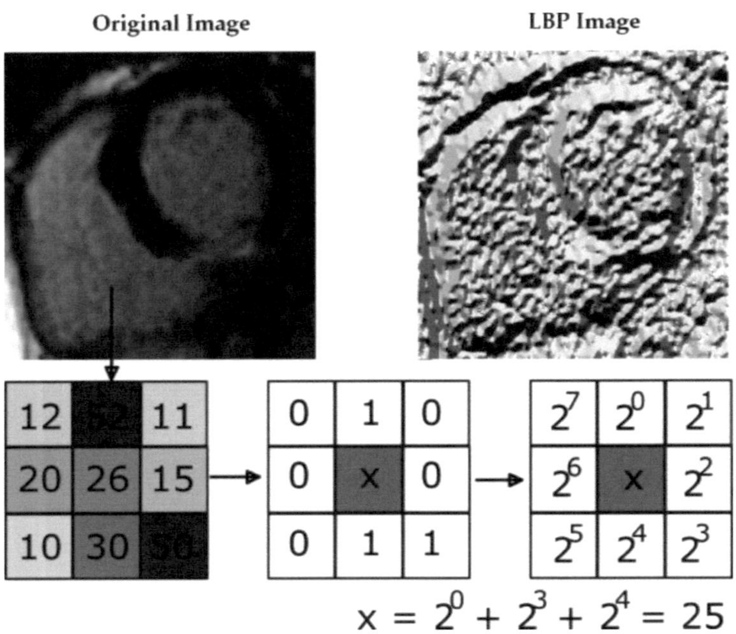

Figure 11. Computation of a basic local binary pattern (LBP) image. For each pixel in the original image, its gray-level is compared to the surrounding pixels. A value of unity is assigned to the pixels with gray-level greater than the central pixel, and a value of zero otherwise. Then a binary number is obtained and this value is assigned to the central pixel.

The original LBP descriptor defined for a 3 × 3 patch was extended to include more neighbors by adding two parameters: parameter P that defines the number of neighbors, and radius R that determines the spatial resolution. Quantification at different resolutions can be obtained by varying these two parameters. Enhancement of the discriminatory power of the LBP descriptor can be obtained by adding an image contrast measure that calculates the local variance in the pixel neighborhood. The contrast measure is the difference between the average gray-level of those pixels that have unity value and those with zero value [20, 14]. Rotation invariance is achieved by performing a bit-wise shift operation on the binary pattern P-1 times and assigning the LBP value that is the smallest. It has been shown by Unay et al. [86] that rotation-invariant LBP is robust against some common MRI artifacts. Their results show that

LBP is robust to image inhomogeneity even at 40% of intensity variations. An extension of the LBP operator on three orthogonal planes, known as LBP-TOP, was proposed by Zhao et al. [87] and successfully applied to the entire brain for 3D texture classification of attention-deficit/hyperactivity disorders [88].

2.4.2. Model-based methods

Texture methods based in models attempt to represent texture by the use of a generative image model (fractals), or a stochastic model. Parameters of the model are then calculated and used for texture analysis. The computational complexity involved in the estimation of features based in models make them less popular than the previously described methods [70].

2.4.2.1 Autoregressive models

The autoregressive models assume a local interaction between the image pixels by considering the pixel gray-level as a weighted sum of its neighbors. Using the autoregressive model involves identifying the model parameters for a given image region and then using them for texture classification [89]. In the study by Holli et al. [40], significant differences were found especially for features derived from the autoregressive model when comparing brain hemispheres in controls and patients with mild traumatic injury. Application of the autoregressive model in different MRI organs was also found beneficial when used in combination with features derived from other methods [4, 64, 90, 91].

2.4.2.2 Fractal models

Fractal models describe objects that have high degree of irregularity. The central concept of fractal models is the property of self-similarity, which is the property of an object to be decomposed into smaller similar copies of itself. Fractal analysis methods provide a statistical measure that reflects pattern changes as a function scale by defining a parameter called fractal dimension. The fractal dimension describes the disorder of an object numerically; the higher the dimension, the more complicated the object. The fractal dimension is often estimated by box counting, a procedure that overlays the image with grids of decreasing size in order to capture the contour of relevant texture. Another approach treats the image as a textured surface by plotting the gray-levels at each x and y position in the z plane [69, 89, 92]. Fractal models have been successfully used especially for segmentation of brain tissues and lesions [72, 93], and for prostate tissue classification in combinations with other methods [26, 94]. For brain tumor evaluation, Yang et al. [63] achieved slightly better results using fractals in comparison with other methods such as LBP, the co-occurrence matrix, and the run-length matrix.

2.4.3. Transform methods

Methods based on image transformation produce an image in a space whose coordinate system is related to texture characteristics, such as frequency content or spatial resolution. Gabor filters provide better spatial localization compared to the Fourier transform, but their usefulness is limited in practice because there is no single filter resolution at which a spatial structure can be localized [70]. In [93], they implemented Gabor features for brain tumor segmentation but the performance was poorer than obtained with fractals and intensity methods, and even combining Gabor features with other methods did not improve the performance. In [95], the co-occurrence matrix features outperformed the Gabor features for 3D classification of brain tumors.

2.4.3.1 The wavelet transform method

The wavelet transform is a technique that analyzes the frequency content of an image within different scales and frequency directions. The frequency is directly proportional to the gray-level variations within the image. Wavelet coefficients corresponding to different frequency scales and directions can be obtained to describe a given image. Wavelet coefficients are associated to each pixel in an image to characterize the frequency content at that point over different scales [3, 89]. **Figure 12** shows an example of a wavelet transform applied to an image at different scales.

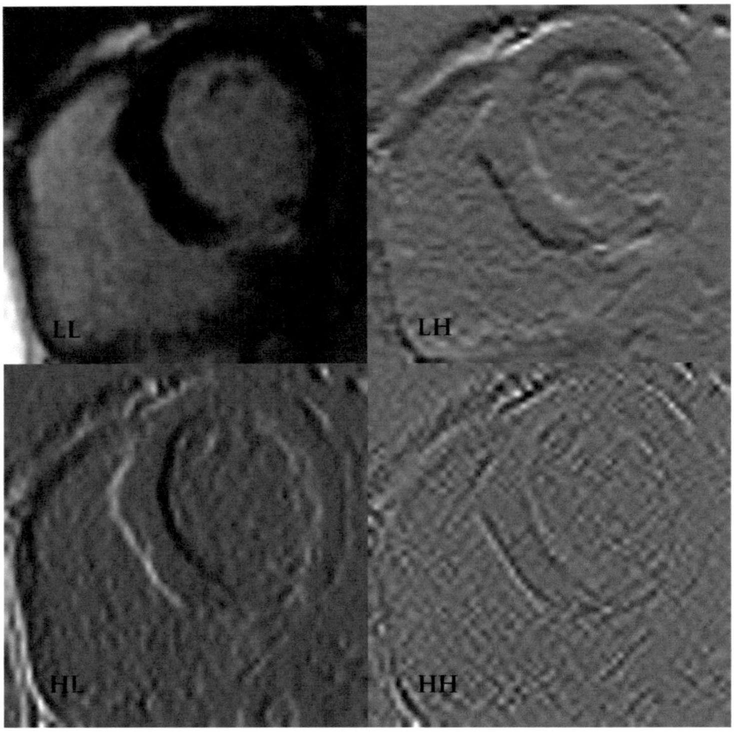

Figure 12. Wavelet transform of a cardiac MR image at one-scale decomposition. The high-high (HH) subimage represents diagonal high frequencies, high-low (HL) extracts the horizontal high frequencies, low-high (LH) vertical high frequencies, and the image low-low (LL) represents the lowest frequencies.

http://dx.doi.org/10.5772/64641

Wavelet transform methods are popular because they offer some advantages, such as: variation of the spatial resolution to represent textures at the most appropriate scale, and the wide range of choices for the wavelet function that can be adjusted for specific applications [70]. Wavelet-derived texture features have high discriminatory power and usually provide better classification than other methods as has been shown for assessment of mild traumatic brain injury [40], knee tissue discrimination [16], and for classification of foam phantoms [18]. It was also demonstrated that wavelet texture features are less sensitive to changes in the MRI acquisition protocol [18]. In some studies the wavelet transform has been used as a preprocessing method to enhance texture appearance by selecting the sub-band with the maximum variance [96, 97]. Features derived from other methods can be extracted from these preprocessed images. Other approaches applied the wavelet transform over previously computed texture maps [10, 85].

2.4.4. 3D texture analysis

Feature extraction methods were first proposed for 2D texture analysis. The advantage of the volumetric nature of MRI datasets can be obtained by extending the original methods to 3D. A simple approach to capture volumetric information is to compute 2D features in all MRI slices and then average these values, as done by Assefa et al. [49], but in this case the gray-level distributions in the third dimension are not taken into account. Nevertheless, it has been shown that even this simple averaging method outperforms the typical 2D approach where only one slice is analyzed [98]. The extension of 2D approaches to 3D is not straightforward as factors such as translation and scaling become more complex. A review of 3D feature extraction methods is presented in [52]. Compared with 2D texture analysis, 3D approaches increase the dimensionality and the information captured from the image, thus improving the discrimination power [44, 99–101]. Implementation of 4D texture analysis is possible by including the temporal dimension available in some MRI datasets. Notable results were observed for discrimination of benign and malignant breast lesions [102] and for localization and segmentation of the heart [103] using the 4D spatio-temporal approach.

2.4.5. Feature extraction tools

The widely used software package MaZda (Institute of Electronics, Technical University of Lodz, Lodz, Poland) [104] is freely available and allows computation of texture features based on co-occurrence matrix, run-length matrix, gradient matrix, autoregressive model, and the Haar wavelet transform. MATLAB (MathWorks Inc., Natick, MA) toolboxes can also be found for texture feature extraction, like the one provided by Vallières et al. [55][2] that allows computation of features based on four matrix methods, and the implementation of the local binary pattern operator provided by Ojala et al. [84][3].

[2] Available from https://github.com/mvallieres/radiomics

[3] Available from http://www.cse.oulu.fi/CMV/Downloads/LBPSoftware

2.5. Feature selection

The vast variety of feature extraction methods for texture analysis allows us to obtain a myriad of features. This generates a problem, because the more features we have, the more complex the classification model becomes. The computed features have different discrimination power depending on the application. Redundant or irrelevant features hinder the classification performance and can yield issues of dimensionality. This phenomenon arises when dealing with a high-dimensional feature space. The classification performance decreases when more features are added to the model. Feature selection is the process to choose the most relevant features for a specific application. Reducing the number of features speeds up the testing of new data and makes the classification problem easier to understand, but the main benefit is the increase of classification performance [105, 106]. While methods like principal component analysis (PCA) or linear discriminant analysis (LDA) are used for feature reduction [23, 56], they are not considered as feature selection methods since they still require computation of all the original features [107].

2.5.1. Filter methods

A straightforward approach to find the most discriminative features, or the combination of features that yields the best classification, is to perform an exhaustive search as done by [26, 33, 108]. In the exhaustive search method, all possible combinations of features are tested as input to a classifier and those that yield the best discrimination are selected. The problem with this method is that it becomes tremendously expensive to compute when the feature space is very high. Filter feature selection methods make use of a certain parameter to measure the discriminatory power. For example, typical statistical methods, such as the Mann-Whitney U-test, can be used to find and select features with statistical significance [64]. The Fisher coefficient defines the ratio of between-class variances to within-class variances and it is a popular filter method found in the literature [21, 40, 47, 109–111]. However, it was claimed that the Fisher technique generates highly correlated features with the same discriminatory power. Another method that relies on both the probability of classification error (POE) and the average correlation coefficient (ACC) was reported to perform better than the Fisher method for classification of knee joint tissues [16]. Filter methods rank the features according to the measuring parameter and usually a predefined number of features is selected, e.g. 5 or 10, for future classification. The Fisher and POE/ACC feature selection methods are implemented in the B11 module which is part of the MaZda software (Institute of Electronics, Technical University of Lodz, Lodz, Poland) [104].

2.5.2. Wrapper methods

The main drawback of the filter methods is that feature selection is based on the intrinsic information of the training data and does not consider the predictive capability of a certain subset of features. Wrapper methods take advantage of a classification algorithm and search the subset of features that provides optimal classification performance. The quality of the selected subset of features depends fundamentally on the search algorithm used. We men-

http://dx.doi.org/10.5772/64641

tioned earlier that an exhaustive search is not feasible for high dimensional datasets, so an algorithm that uses some type of search strategy has to be chosen. Genetic search algorithms have been effectively applied for brain tumor classification [95, 97] and mammogram lesions [98]. Another search algorithm, the recursive feature elimination (RFE), ranks the features by recursively training a classifier and removing the feature with the smallest ranking score and selecting the subset of features that yields the best classification. Any classifier can be used in conjunction with the RFE to compute the feature scores. The feature selection technique known as recursive feature elimination-support vector machine (RFE-SVM), first proposed for gene selection in cancer classification [112], has gained major attention for selecting texture features due to its good performance over other methods [113], and in MRI was particularly used for brain tumor classification [1, 4].

2.6. Classification

The main goal in texture analysis applications is the classification of different tissues and lesions to automate or aid the diagnosis decision. The results of a texture-based classification method can be later used to partition new images into regions, an approach known as texture-based segmentation [70]. Simple statistical methods can be used to determine the texture features with statistical significance for discrimination of two or more classes. However, following the feature selection step described in the previous section, we focus on more complex classification algorithms that make use of proper combination of features to achieve the highest discrimination. The feature selection and classification steps are not specific for texture analysis, so instead of providing a full description of the existing methods, we briefly describe the two classifiers mostly used in MRI texture analysis applications, which are artificial neural networks (ANN) and support vector machines (SVM).

2.6.1. Artificial neural networks

Artificial neural networks (ANN) simulate the way the human brain processes information by implementing nodes and inter-connections. The ANN discrimination power depends on the density and complexity of these interconnections [114]. Applications of ANNs in MRI texture analysis include classification of: brain tumors [23, 115], multiple sclerosis lesions [109], Alzheimer's disease [111], and breast [102] and knee lesions [16]. While ANNs perform well in most applications, their popularity decreased in the past years due to the introduction of the support vector machine (SVM), which is computationally cheaper and provides similar or even better performance than ANNs [114].

2.6.2. Support vector machines

The SVM maps the input space to a higher dimension via a kernel function to find a hyperplane that will result in maximal discrimination. Here, a kernel is a matrix that encodes the similarities between samples that can be used to achieve discrimination between classes that are not linearly separable [114]. In [4], they demonstrated better performance of the SVM classifier over ANN for differentiation of benign and malignant brain tumors. SVMs were also applied for brain tumor classification in [1, 116]. Other applications of SVMs include the staging of liver fibrosis [33], detection of prostate [26], assessment of osteoarthritis [117], classification of cervical cancer [118], mammogram lesions [98], and Parkinson disease [73].

2.6.3. Classification results

Important considerations have to be made when reporting classification results. To avoid overestimated values, it is always recommended to separate the data into training and validation sets so that results on new data can be reported. When the dataset is sparse, resampling approaches like cross-validation or bootstrapping are recommended. For unbalanced data, i.e., data containing more normal than abnormal tissues, it is suggested to report results using the area under the curve (AUC) of the receiver operating characteristic (ROC) instead of the overall accuracy or misclassification rate [114]. Feature vector standardization is recommended and required for some classification methods to work accurately and to improve accuracy in some cases [16].

3. Summary

In this chapter, we reviewed the literature regarding the application of texture analysis in MRI. This chapter was organized and focused on the six steps that define the texture analysis process: MRI acquisition, ROI definition, ROI preprocessing, feature extraction, feature selection, and classification. Our main goal was to provide a condensed reference of the state of the art and especially to make readers aware about important considerations to be made for future applications in order to implement MRI texture analysis into clinical practice. Since many parameters can vary in each step, it is impossible to give a definite guideline of what needs to be used, while each choice has to be made in view of the specific application. The clinical applicability relies on the reproducibility of the methods regarding the scanner and acquisition parameters. Therefore, it is necessary to execute more multicenter studies combining different acquisition protocols and applying appropriate preprocessing steps to ensure that texture features describe the actual image characteristics and are not biased by other factors. Regarding the ROI definition step, it is recommended to carry out studies using automatic methods to guarantee user independence. Finally, we suggest to compute as many texture features as possible and to take advantage of powerful feature selection and classification techniques to achieve the highest performance.

Acknowledgements

This work was supported in part by the Spanish Ministerio de Economía y Competitividad (MINECO) FEDER funds under grant BFU2015-64380-C2-2-R, by Instituto de Salud Carlos III and FEDER funds under grants FIS PI14/00271 and PIE15/00013 and by the Generalitat Valenciana under grant PROMETEO/2013/007. The first author, Andrés Larroza, was supported by grant FPU12/01140 from the Spanish Ministerio de Educación, Cultura y Deporte (MECD).

Author details

Andrés Larroza[1], Vicente Bodí[1] and David Moratal[2*]

*Address all correspondence to: dmoratal@eln.upv.es

1 Department of Medicine, Universitat de València, Valencia, Spain

2 Center for Biomaterials and Tissue Engineering, Universitat Politècnica de València, Valencia, Spain

References

[1] Larroza A, Moratal D, Paredes-Sánchez A, Soria-Olivas E, Chust ML, Arribas LA, Arana E. Support vector machine classification of brain metastasis and radiation necrosis based on texture analysis in MRI. Journal of Magnetic Resonance Imaging. 2015;42(5): 1362–1368. DOI: 10.1002/jmri.24913

[2] Castellano G, Bonilha L, Li LM, Cendes F. Texture analysis of medical images. Clinical Radiology. 2004;59:1061–1069. DOI: 10.1016/j.crad.2004.07.008

[3] Materka A. What is the texture? In: Hajek M, Dezortova M, Materka A, Lerski R, Editors. Texture Analysis for Magnetic Resonance Imaging. 1st Ed. Prague, Czech Republic: Med4publishing; 2006. p. 11–40.

[4] Juntu J, Sijbers J, De Backer S, Rajan J, Van Dyck D. Machine learning study of several classifiers trained with texture analysis features to differentiate benign from malignant soft-tissue tumors in T1-MRI images. Journal of Magnetic Resonance Imaging. 2010;31(3):680–689. DOI: 10.1002/jmri.22095

[5] Zacharaki EI, Wang S, Chawla S, Soo Yoo D, Wolf R, Melhem ER, Davatzikos C. Classification of brain tumor type and grade using MRI texture and shape in a machine learning scheme. Magnetic Resonance in Medicine. 2009;62(6):1609–1618. DOI: 10.1002/mrm.22147

[6] De Oliveira MS, Balthazar ML, D'Abreu A, Yasuda CL, Damasceno BP, Cendes F, Castellano G. MR imaging texture analysis of the corpus callosum and thalamus in amnestic mild cognitive impairment and mild Alzheimer disease. American Journal of Neuroradiology. 2011;32(1):60–66. DOI: 10.3174/ajnr.A2232

[7] Santos TA, Maistro CE, Silva CB, Oliveira MS, Franca MC, Castellano G. MRI texture analysis reveals bulbar abnormalities in Friedreich ataxia. American Journal of Neuroradiology. 2015;36(12):2214–2218. DOI: 10.3174/ajnr.A4455

[8] Karimaghaloo Z, Rivaz H, Arnold DL, Collins DL, Arbel T. Temporal hierarchical adaptive texture CRF for automatic detection of gadolinium-enhancing multiple sclerosis lesions in brain MRI. IEEE Transactions on Medical Imaging. 2015;34(6):1227–1241. DOI: 10.1109/TMI.2014.2382561

[9] Iftekharuddin KM, Ahmed S, Hossen J. Multiresolution texture models for brain tumor segmentation in MRI. In: 33rd Annual International Conference of the IEEE Engineering in Medicine and Biology Society, IEEE, Boston, Massachusetts, USA; 2011. p. 6985–6988. DOI: 10.1109/IEMBS.2011.6091766

[10] Yao J, Chen J, Chow C. Breast tumor analysis in dynamic contrast enhanced MRI using texture features and Wavelet transform. IEEE Journal of Selected Topics in Signal Processing. 2009;3(1):94–100. DOI: 10.1109/JSTSP.2008.2011110

[11] Jirák D, Dezortová M, Taimr P, Hájek M. Texture analysis of human liver. Journal of Magnetic Resonance Imaging. 2002;15(1):68–74. DOI: 10.1002/jmri.10042 68

[12] Ghose S, Oliver A, Martí R, Lladó X, Freixenet J, Vilanova JC, Meriaudeau F. Prostate segmentation with local binary patterns guided active appearance models. In: Proceedings of SPIE 7962, Medical Imaging: Image Processing, 796218, SPIE, Lake Buena Vista, Florida, USA; 2011. DOI: 10.1117/12.877955

[13] Eftestøl T, Maløy F, Engan K, Kotu LP, Woie L, Ørn S. A texture-based probability mapping for localisation of clinically important cardiac segments in the myocardium in cardiac magnetic resonance images from myocardial infarction patients. In: IEEE International Conference on Image Processing (ICIP), IEEE, Paris, France; 2014. p. 2227–2231. DOI: 10.1109/ICIP.2014.7025451

[14] Kotu LP, Engan K, Eftestøl T, Woie L, Ørn S, Katsaggelos AK. Local binary patterns used on cardiac MRI to classify high and low risk patient groups. In: Proceedings of the 20th European Signal Processing Conference (EUSIPCO), IEEE, Bucharest, Romania; 2012. p. 2586–2590.

[15] Schad LR, Lundervold A. Influence of resolution and signal to noise ratio on MR image texture. In: Hajek M, Dezortova M, Materka A, Lerski R, Editors. Texture Analysis for Magnetic Resonance Imaging. 1st ed. Prague, Czech Republic: Med4publishing; 2006. p. 127–147.

[16] Mayerhoefer ME, Breitenseher MJ, Kramer J, Aigner N, Hofmann S, Materka A. Texture analysis for tissue discrimination on T1-weighted MR images of the knee joint in a multicenter study: Transferability of texture features and comparison of feature selection methods and classifiers. Journal of Magnetic Resonance Imaging. 2005;22(5): 674–680.

[17] Schad LR. Problems in texture analysis with magnetic resonance imaging. Dialogues in Clinical Neuroscience. 2004;6(2):235–242.

[18] Waugh SA, Lerski RA, Bidaut L, Thompson AM. The influence of field strength and different clinical breast MRI protocols on the outcome of texture analysis using foam phantoms. Medical Physics. 2011;38(9):5058–5066. DOI: 10.1118/1.3622605

[19] Tiwari P, Prasanna P, Rogers L, Wolansky L, Badve C, Sloan A, Cohen M, Madabhushi A. Texture descriptors to distinguish radiation necrosis from recurrent brain tumors on multi-parametric MRI. In: Aylward S, Hadjiiski LM, Editors. SPIE Medical Imaging, SPIE, San Diego, California, USA; 2014. vol. 9035. p. 90352B. DOI: 10.1117/12.2043969

[20] Oppedal K, Eftestøl T, Engan K, Beyer MK, Aarsland D. Classifying dementia using local binary patterns from different regions in magnetic resonance images. International Journal of Biomedical Imaging. 2015;2015:1-14. DOI: 10.1155/2015/572567

[21] Herlidou-Même S, Constans JM, Carsin B, Olivie D, Eliat PA, Nadal-Desbarats L, Gondry C, Le Rumeur E, Idy-Peretti I, de Certaines JD. MRI texture analysis on texture test objects, normal brain and intracranial tumors. Magnetic Resonance Imaging. 2003;21(9):989–993.

[22] Fruehwald-Pallamar J, Hesselink J, Mafee M, Holzer-Fruehwald L, Czerny C, Mayerhoefer M. Texture-based analysis of 100 MR examinations of head and neck tumors – is it possible to discriminate between benign and malignant masses in a multicenter trial? Fortschr Röntgenstr. 2016;188(2):195–202. DOI: 10.1055/s-0041-106066

[23] Orphanidou-Vlachou E, Vlachos N, Davies NP, Arvanitis TN, Grundy RG, Peet AC. Texture analysis of T1- and T2-weighted MR images and use of probabilistic neural network to discriminate posterior fossa tumours in children. NMR in Biomedicine. 2014;27(6):632–639. DOI: 10.1002/nbm.3099

[24] Brynolfsson P, Nilsson D, Henriksson R, Hauksson J, Karlsson M, Garpebring A, Birgander R, Trygg J, Nyholm T, Asklund T. ADC texture—an imaging biomarker for high-grade glioma? Medical Physics. 2014;41(10):101903. DOI: 10.1118/1.4894812

[25] Foroutan P, Kreahling JM, Morse DL, Grove O, Lloyd MC, Reed D, Raghavan M, Altiok S, Martinez GV, Gillies RJ. Diffusion MRI and novel texture analysis in osteosarcoma xenotransplants predicts response to anti-checkpoint therapy. PLoS One. 2013;8(12):e82875. DOI: 10.1371/journal.pone.0082875

[26] Khalvati F, Wong A, Haider MA. Automated prostate cancer detection via comprehensive multi-parametric magnetic resonance imaging texture feature models. BMC Medical Imaging. 2015;15:27. DOI: 10.1186/s12880-015-0069-9

[27] Jirák D, Dezortová M, Hájek M. Phantoms for texture analysis of MR images. Long-term and multi-center study. Medical Physics. 2004;31(3):616–622.

[28] Mayerhoefer ME, Szomolanyi P, Jirak D, Materka A, Trattnig S. Effects of MRI acquisition parameter variations and protocol heterogeneity on the results of texture analysis

and pattern discrimination: An application-oriented study. Medical Physics. 2009;36(4): 1236–1243. DOI: 10.1118/1.3081408

[29] Jirák D, Dezortova M, Hajek M. Phantoms for texture analysis of MR images. In: Hajek M, Dezortova M, Materka A, Lerski R, Editors. Texture Analysis for Magnetic Resonance Imaging. 1st ed. Prague, Czech Republic: Med4publishing; 2006. p. 113–124.

[30] Tameem HZ, Selva LE, Sinha US. Texture measure from low resolution MR images to determine trabecular bone integrity in osteoporosis. In: 29th Annual International Conference of the IEEE on Engineering in Medicine and Biology Society, EMBS 2007, IEEE, Lyon, France; 2007. p. 2027–2030. DOI: 10.1109/IEMBS.2007.4352717

[31] Savio SJ, Harrison LCV, Luukkaala T, Heinonen T, Dastidar P, Soimakallio S, Eskola HJ. Effect of slice thickness on brain magnetic resonance image texture analysis. Biomedical Engineering Online. 2010;9:60. DOI: 10.1186/1475-925X-9-60

[32] Bradley WG. Pros and cons of 3 Tesla MRI. Journal of the American College of Radiology. 2009;5(8):871–878. DOI: 10.1016/j.jacr.2008.02.005

[33] Zhang X, Gao X, Liu BJ, Ma K, Yan W, Liling L, Yuhong H, Fujita H. Effective staging of fibrosis by the selected texture features of liver: Which one is better, CT or MR imaging? Computerized Medical Imaging and Graphics. 2015;46:227–236. DOI: 10.1016/j.compmedimag.2015.09.003

[34] Giger M, Li H, Lan L, Abe H, Newstead G. Quantitative MRI phenotyping of breast cancer across molecular classification subtypes. In: Fujita H, Hara T, Muramatsu C, Editors. Breast Imaging. Volume 8539 of the series Lecture Notes in Computer Science. Springer, Switzerland; 2014. p. 195–200. DOI: 10.1007/978-3-319-07887-8_28

[35] Sanz-Cortes M, Figueras F, Bonet-Carne E, Padilla N, Tenorio V, Bargalló N, Amat-Roldn I, Gratacós E. Fetal brain MRI texture analysis identifies different microstructural patterns in adequate and small for gestational age fetuses at term. Fetal Diagnosis and Therapy. 2013;33(2):122–129. DOI: 10.1159/000346566

[36] Harrison LCV, Nikander R, Sikiö M, Luukkaala T, Helminen MT, Ryymin P, Soimakallio S, Eskola HJ, Dastidar P, Sievänen H. MRI texture analysis of femoral neck: Detection of exercise load-associated differences in trabecular bone. Journal of Magnetic Resonance Imaging. 2011;34(6):1359–1366. DOI: 10.1002/jmri.22751

[37] Shi Z, Yang Z, Zhang G, Cui G, Xiong X, Liang Z, Lu H. Characterization of texture features of bladder carcinoma and the bladder wall on MRI: Initial experience. Academic Radiology. 2013;20(8):930–938. DOI: 10.1016/j.acra.2013.03.011

[38] Loizou CP, Petroudi S, Seimenis I, Pantziaris M, Pattichis CS. Quantitative texture analysis of brain white matter lesions derived from T2-weighted MR images in MS patients with clinically isolated syndrome. Journal of Neuroradiology. 2015;42(2):99–114. DOI: 10.1016/j.neurad.2014.05.006

[39] Liu H, Shao Y, Guo D, Zheng Y, Zhao Z, Qiu T. Cirrhosis classification based on texture classification of random features. Computational and Mathematical Methods in Medicine. 2014;2014:536308. DOI: 10.1155/2014/536308

[40] Holli KK, Harrison L, Dastidar P, Wäljas M, Liimatainen S, Luukkaala T, Ohman J, Soimakallio S, Eskola H. Texture analysis of MR images of patients with mild traumatic brain injury. BMC Medical Imaging. 2010;10:8. DOI: 10.1186/1471-2342-10-8

[41] Karimaghaloo Z, Rivaz H, Arnold DL, Collins DL, Arbel T. Adaptive voxel, texture and temporal conditional random fields for detection of Gad-enhancing multiple sclerosis lesions in brain MRI. In: Medical Image Computing and Computer-Assisted Intervention-MICCAI 2013, Springer, Nagoya, Japan; 2013. p. 543–550. DOI: 10.1007/978-3-642-40760-4_68

[42] Vignati A, Mazzetti S, Giannini V, Russo F, Bollito E, Porpiglia F, Stasi M, Regge D. Texture features on T2-weighted magnetic resonance imaging: New potential biomarkers for prostate cancer aggressiveness. Physics in Medicine and Biology. 2015;60(7): 2685–2701. DOI: 10.1088/0031-9155/60/7/2685

[43] Mayerhoefer ME, Stelzeneder D, Bachbauer W, Welsch GH, Mamisch TC, Szczypinski P, et al. Quantitative analysis of lumbar intervertebral disc abnormalities at 3.0 Tesla: Value of T(2) texture features and geometric parameters. NMR in Biomedicine. 2012;25(6):866–872. DOI: 10.1002/nbm.1803

[44] Chen W, Giger ML, Li H, Bick U, Newstead GM. Volumetric texture analysis of breast lesions on contrast-enhanced magnetic resonance images. Magnetic Resonance in Medicine. 2007;58(3):562–571.

[45] Materka A. Statistical methods. In: Hajek M, Dezortova M, Materka A, Lerski R, Editors. Texture Analysis for Magnetic Resonance Imaging. 1st ed. Prague, Czech Republic: Med4publishing; 2006. p. 79–103.

[46] Sikiö M, Harrison L, Eskola H. The effect of region of interest size on textural parameters. A study with clinical magnetic resonance images and artificial noise images. In: 9th International Symposium on Image and Signal Processing and Analysis (ISPA), IEEE, Zagreb, Croatia; 2015. p. 149–153. DOI: 10.1109/ISPA. 2015.7306049

[47] Antel SB, Collins DL, Bernasconi N, Andermann F, Shinghal R, Kearney RE, Arnold DL, Bernasconi A. Automated detection of focal cortical dysplasia lesions using computational models of their MRI characteristics and texture analysis. Neuroimage. 2003;19(4):1748–1759. DOI: 10.1016/S1053-8119(03)00226-X

[48] Kjaer L, Ring P, Thomsen C, Henriksen O. Texture analysis in quantitative MR imaging. Tissue characterisation of normal brain and intracranial tumours at 1.5 T. Acta Radiologica. 1995;36(2):127–135.

[49] Assefa D, Keller H, Ménard C, Laperriere N, Ferrari RJ, Yeung I. Robust texture features for response monitoring of glioblastoma multiforme on T1-

weighted and T2-FLAIR MR images: A preliminary investigation in terms of identification and segmentation. Medical Physics. 2010;37(4):1722–1736. DOI: 10.1118/1.3357289

[50] Chen X, Wei X, Zhang Z, Yang R, Zhu Y, Jiang X. Differentiation of true-progression from pseudoprogression in glioblastoma treated with radiation therapy and concomitant temozolomide by GLCM texture analysis of conventional MRI. Clinical Imaging. 2015;39(5):775–780. DOI: 10.1016/j.clinimag.2015.04.003

[51] Mayerhoefer ME, Szomolanyi P, Jirak D, Berg A, Materka A, Dirisamer A, Trattnig S. Effects of magnetic resonance image interpolation on the results of texture-based pattern classification: A phantom study. Investigative Radiology. 2009;44(7):405–411. DOI: 10.1097/RLI.0b013e3181a50a66

[52] Depeursinge A, Foncubierta-Rodriguez A, Van De Ville D, Müller H. Three-dimensional solid texture analysis in biomedical imaging: Review and opportunities. Medical Image Analysis. 2014;18(51):176–196. DOI: 10.1016/j.media.2013.10.005

[53] Materka A, Strzelecki M, Lerski R, Schad L. Evaluation of texture features of test objects for magnetic resonance imaging. In: Pietikainen M, Editor. Infotech Oulu Workshop on Texture Analysis in Machine Vision. Infotech, Oulu, Finland; 1999. p. 13–19.

[54] Collewet G, Strzelecki M, Mariette F. Influence of MRI acquisition protocols and image intensity normalization methods on texture classification. Magnetic Resonance Imaging. 2004;22(1):81–91. DOI: 10.1016/j.mri.2003.09.001

[55] Vallières M, Freeman CR, Skamene SR, El Naqa I. A radiomics model from joint FDG-PET and MRI texture features for the prediction of lung metastases in soft-tissue sarcomas of the extremities. Physics in Medicine and Biology. 2015;60(14):5471–5496. DOI: 10.1088/0031-9155/60/14/5471

[56] Thornhill RE, Golfam M, Sheikh A, Cron GO, White EA, Werier J, Schweitzer ME, Di Primio G. Differentiation of lipoma from liposarcoma on MRI using texture and shape analysis. Academic Radiology. 2014;21(9):1185–1194. DOI: 10.1016/j.acra.2014.04.005

[57] Kölhi P, Järnstedt J, Sikiö M, Viik J, Dastidar P, Peltomäki T, Eskola H. A texture analysis method for MR images of airway dilator muscles: A feasibility study. Dentomaxillofacial Radiology. 2014;43(5):20130403. DOI: 10.1259/dmfr.20130403

[58] Loizou CP, Pantziaris M, Seimenis I, Pattichis CS. Brain MR image normalization in texture analysis of multiple sclerosis. In: 9th International Conference on Information Technology and Applications in Biomedicine, 2009, ITAB 2009, IEEE, Larnaca, Cyprus; 2009. p. 1–5. DOI: 10.1109/ITAB.2009.5394331

[59] Materka A, Strzelecki M. On the importance of MRI nonuniformity correction for texture analysis. In: Conference Proceedings of Signal Processing: Algorithms, Architectures, Arrangements, and Applications (SPA), IEEE, Poznan, Poland; 2013. p. 118–123.

[60] Belaroussi B, Milles J, Carme S, Zhu YM, Benoit-Cattin H. Intensity non-uniformity correction in MRI: Existing methods and their validation. Medical Image Analysis. 2006;10(2):234–246. DOI: 10.1016/j.media.2005.09.004

[61] Prasanna P, Tiwari P, Madabhushi A. Co-occurrence of local anisotropic gradient orientations (CoLlAGe): Distinguishing tumor confounders and molecular subtypes on MRI. In: Medical Image Computing and Computer-Assisted Intervention-MICCAI 2014, Springer, Boston, MA, USA; 2014. p. 73–78. DOI: 10.1007/978-3-319-10443-0_10

[62] Zhang Y, Traboulsee A, Zhao Y, Metz LM, Li DK. Texture analysis differentiates persistent and transient T1 black holes at acute onset in multiple sclerosis: A preliminary study. Multiple Sclerosis Journal. 2011;17(5):532–540. DOI: 10.1177/1352458510395981

[63] Yang D, Rao G, Martinez J, Veeraraghavan A, Rao A. Evaluation of tumor-derived MRI-texture features for discrimination of molecular subtypes and prediction of 12-month survival status in glioblastoma. Medical Physics. 2015;42(11):6725–6735. DOI: 10.1118/1.4934373

[64] Chuah TK, Van Reeth E, Sheah K, Poh CL. Texture analysis of bone marrow in knee MRI for classification of subjects with bone marrow lesion – data from the osteoarthritis initiative. Magnetic Resonance Imaging. 2013;31(6):930–938. DOI: 10.1016/j.mri.2013.01.014

[65] Sled JG, Zijdenbos AP, Evans AC. A nonparametric method for automatic correction of intensity nonuniformity in MRI data. IEEE Transactions on Medical Imaging. 1998;17(1):87–97. DOI: 10.1109/42.668698

[66] Gibbs P, Turnbull LW. Textural analysis of contrast-enhanced MR images of the breast. Magnetic Resonance in Medicine. 2003;50(1):92–98. DOI: 10.1002/mrm.10496

[67] Ahmed A, Gibbs P, Pickles M, Turnbull L. Texture analysis in assessment and prediction of chemotherapy response in breast cancer. Journal of Magnetic Resonance Imaging. 2013;38(1):89–101. DOI: 10.1002/jmri.23971

[68] Mahmoud-Ghoneim D, Alkaabi MK, de Certaines JD, Goettsche FM. The impact of image dynamic range on texture classification of brain white matter. BMC Medical Imaging. 2008;8:18. DOI: 10.1186/1471-2342-8-18

[69] Nailon H. Texture analysis methods for medical image characterisation. In: Mao Y, Editor. Biomedical Imaging. InTech, Rijeka, Croatia; 2010. p. 75-100. DOI: 10.5772/8912

[70] Materka A. Texture analysis methodologies for magnetic resonance imaging. Dialogues in Clinical Neuroscience. 2004;6:243–250.

[71] Ain Q, Jaffar MA, Choi TS. Fuzzy anisotropic diffusion based segmentation and texture based ensemble classification of brain tumor. Applied Soft Computing. 2014;21:330–340. DOI: 10.1016/j.asoc.2014.03.019

[72] Ahmed S, Iftekharuddin KM, Vossough A. Efficacy of texture, shape, and intensity feature fusion for posterior-fossa tumor segmentation in MRI. IEEE Transactions on Information Technology in Biomedicine. 2011;15(2):206–213. DOI: 10.1109/TITB.2011.2104376

[73] Mohanty DR, Mishra SK. MRI classification of Parkinson's disease using SVM and texture features. In: Proceedings of the Second International Conference on Computer and Communication Technologies, Springer, India; 2016. p. 357–364. DOI: 10.1007/978-81-322-2523-2_34

[74] Haralick RM, Shanmugam K, Dinstein I. Textural features for image classification. IEEE Transactions on Systems, Man, and Cybernetics SMC-3. 1973;6:610–621. DOI: 10.1109/TSMC.1973.4309314

[75] Haralick RM. Statistical and structural approaches to texture. Proceedings of the IEEE. 1979;67(5):786–804. DOI: 10.1109/PROC.1979.11328

[76] Wibmer A, Hricak H, Gondo T, Matsumoto K, Veeraraghavan H, Fehr D, Zheng J, Goldman D, Moskowitz C, Fine SW, Reuter VE, Eastham J, Sala E, Vargas HA. Haralick texture analysis of prostate MRI: Utility for differentiating non-cancerous prostate from prostate cancer and differentiating prostate cancers with different Gleason scores. European Radiology. 2015;25(10):2840–2850. DOI: 10.1007/s00330-015-3701-8

[77] Kovalev V, Kruggel F. Texture anisotropy of the brain's white matter as revealed by anatomical MRI. IEEE Transactions in Medical Imaging. 2007;26(5):678–685. DOI: 10.1109/TMI.2007.895481

[78] Suoranta S, Holli-Helenius K, Koskenkorva P, Niskanen E, Könönen M, Äikiä M, Eskola H, Kälviaïanen R, Vanninen R. 3D texture analysis reveals imperceptible MRI textural alterations in the thalamus and putamen in progressive myoclonic epilepsy type 1, EPM1. PLoS One. 2013;8(7):e69905. DOI: 10.1371/journal.pone.0069905

[79] House MJ, Bangma SJ, Thomas M, Gan EK, Ayonrinde OT, Adams LA, Olynyk JK, St Pierre TG. Texture-based classification of liver fibrosis using MRI. Journal of Magnetic Resonance Imaging. 2015;41(2):322–328. DOI: 10.1002/jmri.24536

[80] Bonilha L, Kobayashi E, Castellano G, Coelho G, Tinois E, Cendes F, Li LM. Texture analysis of hippocampal sclerosis. Epilepsia. 2003;44(12):1546–1550. DOI: 10.1111/j.0013-9580.2003.27103.x

[81] Boutsikou K, Kostopoulos S, Glotsos D, Cavouras D, Lavdas E, Oikonomou G, Malizos K, Fezoulidis IV, Vlychou M. Texture analysis of articular cartilage traumatic changes in the knee calculated from morphological 3.0 T MR imaging. European Journal of Radiology. 2013;82(8):1266–1272. DOI: 10.1016/j.ejrad.2013.01.023

[82] Galloway MM. Texture analysis using gray level run lengths. Computer Graphics and Image Processing. 1975;4(2):172–179. DOI: 10.1016/S0146-664X(75)80008-6

[83] Loh HH, Leu JG, Luo RC. The analysis of natural textures using run length features. Journal of Magnetic Resonance Imaging. 1988;35(2):323–328. DOI: 10.1109/41.192665

[84] Ojala T, Pietikäinen M, Mäenpää T. A generalized local binary pattern operator for multiresolution gray scale and rotation invariant texture classification. In: Second International Conference ICAPR 2001, Springer, Rio de Janeiro, Brazil; 2001. p. 399–408. DOI: 10.1007/3-540-44732-6_41

[85] Sheethal MS, Kannanm DB, Varghese A, Sobha T. Intelligent classification technique of human brain MRI with Efficient Wavelet based Feature Extraction using Local Binary Pattern. In: International Conference on Control Communication and Computing (ICCC), IEEE, Thiruvananthapuram, India; 2013. p. 368–372. DOI: 10.1109/ICCC.2013.6731681

[86] Unay D, Ekin A, Cetin M, Jasinschi R, Ercil A. Robustness of local binary patterns in brain MR image analysis. In: 29th Annual International Conference on Engineering in Medicine and Biology Society, EMBS 2007, IEEE, Lyon, France; 2007. p. 2098–2101. DOI: 10.1109/IEMBS.2007Arunadevi B, Deepa SN. Texture analysis for 3D classification of brain tumor tissues. Przegląd Elektrotechniczny. 2013;4:342–348. .4352735

[87] Zhao G, Pietikainen M. Dynamic texture recognition using local binary patterns with an application to facial expressions. IEEE Transactions on Pattern Analysis and Machine Intelligence. 2007;29(6):915–928. DOI: 10.1109/TPAMI.2007.1110

[88] Chang C-W, Ho C-C, Chen J-H. ADHD classification by a texture analysis of anatomical brain MRI data. Frontiers in Systems Neuroscience. 2012;6:66. DOI: 10.3389/fnsys.2012.00066

[89] Materka A, Strzelecki M. Texture Analysis Methods: A Review. Institute of Electronics, Technical University of Lodz, Poland; 1998. Vol. 11. p. 1–32.

[90] Skoch A, Jirák D, Vyhnanovská P, Dezortová M, Fendrych P, Rolencová E, Hájek M. Classification of calf muscle MR images by texture analysis. Magnetic Resonance Material in Physics. 2004;16(6):259–267. DOI: 10.1007/s10334-004-0032-1

[91] Wu Z, Matsui O, Kitao A, Kozaka K, Koda W, Kobayashi S, Ryu Y, Minami T, Sanada J, Gabata T. Hepatitis C related chronic liver cirrhosis: Feasibility of texture analysis of MR images for classification of fibrosis stage and necroinflammatory activity grade. PLoS One. 2015;10(3):30118297. DOI: 10.1371/journal.pone.0118297

[92] Alic L, Niessen WJ, Veenland JF. Quantification of heterogeneity as a biomarker in tumor imaging: A systematic review. PLoS One. 2014;9(10):e110300. DOI: 10.1371/journal.pone.0110300

[93] Islam A, Reza SMS, Iftekharuddin KM. Multifractal texture estimation for detection and segmentation of brain tumors. IEEE Transactions on Biomedical Engineering. 2013;60(11):3204–3215. DOI: 10.1109/TBME.2013.2271383

[94] Duda D, Kretowski M, Mathieu R, de Crevoisier R, Bezy-Wendling J. Multi-image texture analysis in classification of prostatic tissues from MRI. Preliminary results. In:

Pietka E, Kawa J, Wieclawek W, Editors. Information Technologies in Biomedicine. Volume 3. Springer International Publishing, Switzerland; 2014. p. 139–150. DOI: 10.1007/978-3-319-06593-9_13

[95] Arunadevi B, Deepa SN. Texture analysis for 3D classification of brain tumor tissues. 30 Przegląd Elektrotechniczny. 2013;4:342–348.

[96] Meenakshi R, Anandhakumar P. Wavelet statistical texture features with orthogonal operators tumour classification in magnetic resonance imaging brain. American Journal of Applied Sciences. 2013;10(10):1154–1159. DOI: 10.3844/ajassp.2013.1154.1159

[97] Sasikala M, Kumaravel N. A wavelet-based optimal texture feature set for classification of brain tumours. Journal of Medical Engineering & Technology. 2008;32(3):198–205. DOI: 10.1080/03091900701455524

[98] Wagner F, Gryanik A, Schulz-Wendtland R, Fasching PA, Wittenberg T. 3D characterization of texture: Evaluation for the potential application in mammographic mass diagnosis. Biomedical Engineering. 2012;57:490–493. DOI: 10.1515/bmt-2012-4240

[99] Kovalev VA, Kruggel F, Gertz HJ, Von Cramon DY. Three-dimensional texture analysis of MRI brain datasets. IEEE Transactions on Medical Imaging. 2001;20(5):424–433. DOI: 10.1109/42.925295

[100] Mahmoud-Ghoneim D, Toussaint G, Constans JM, De Certaines JD. Three dimensional texture analysis in MRI: A preliminary evaluation in gliomas. Magnetic Resonance Imaging. 2003;21(9):983–987. DOI: 10.1016/S0730-725X(03)00201-7

[101] Georgiadis P, Cavouras D, Kalatzis I, Glotsos D, Athanasiadis E, Kostopoulos S, Sifaki K, Malamas M, Nikiforidis G, Solomou E. Enhancing the discrimination accuracy between metastases, gliomas and meningiomas on brain MRI by volumetric textural features and ensemble pattern recognition methods. Magnetic Resonance Imaging. 2009;27(1):120–130. DOI: 10.1016/j.mri.2008.05.017

[102] Woods BJ, Clymer BD, Kurc T, Heverhagen JT, Stevens R, Orsdemir A, Bulan O, Knopp MV. Malignant-lesion segmentation using 4D co-occurrence texture analysis applied to dynamic contrast-enhanced magnetic resonance breast image data. Journal of Magnetic Resonance Imaging. 2007;25(3):495–501. DOI: 10.1002/jmri.20837

[103] Huang J, Huang X, Metaxas D, Axel L. Dynamic texture based heart localization and segmentation in 4-D cardiac images. In: 4th IEEE International Symposium on Biomedical Imaging: From Nano to Macro, IEEE, Arlington, VA; 2007. p. 852–855. DOI: 10.1109/ISBI.2007.356986

[104] Szczypinski PM, Strzelecki M, Materka A, Klepaczko A. MaZda. A software package for image texture analysis. Computer Methods and Programs in Biomedicine. 2009;94(1):66–76. DOI: 10.1016/j.cmpb.2008.08.005

[105] Guyon I, Elisseeff A. An introduction to variable and feature selection. Journal of Machine Learning Research. 2003;3:1157–1182. DOI: 10.1162/153244303322753616

[106] Chu C, Hsu A-L, Chou K-H, Bandettini P, Lin C. Does feature selection improve classification accuracy? Impact of sample size and feature selection on classification using anatomical magnetic resonance images. NeuroImage. 2012;60(1):59–70. DOI: 10.1016/j.neuroimage.2011.11.066

[107] Bhalerao A, Reyes-Aldasoro CC. Volumetric texture description and discriminant feature selection for MRI. Information Processing in Medical Imaging. 2003;18:282–293. DOI: 10.1007/b13239

[108] Boniatis I, Klironomos G, Gatzounis G, Panayiotakis G. Texture-based characterization of pre- and post-operative T2-weighted magnetic resonance signals of the cervical spinal cord in cervical spondylotic myelopathy. In: IEEE International Workshop on Imaging Systems and Techniques, IEEE; 2008. p. 353–356. DOI: 10.1109/IST.2008.4660000

[109] Zhang J, Tong L, Wang L, Li N. Texture analysis of multiple sclerosis: A comparative study. Magnetic Resonance Imaging. 2008;26(8):1160–1166. DOI: 10.1016/j.mri.2008.01.016

[110] Nketiah G, Savio S, Dastidar P, Nikander R, Eskola H, Sievänen H. Detection of exercise load-associated differences in hip muscles by texture analysis. Scandinavian Journal of Medicine & Science in Sports. 2015;25(3):428–434. DOI: 10.1111/sms.12247

[111] Zhang J, Yu C, Jiang G, Liu W, Tong L. 3D texture analysis on MRI images of Alzheimer's disease. Brain Imaging and Behavior. 2012;6(1):61–69. DOI: 10.1007/s11682-011-9142-3

[112] Guyon I, Weston J, Barnhill S, Vapnik V. Gene selection for cancer classification using support vector machines. Machine Learning. 2002;46(1–3):389–422. DOI: 10.1023/A:1012487302797

[113] Fernandez-Lozano C, Seoane JA, Gestal M, Gaunt TR, Dorado J, Campbell C. Texture classification using feature selection and kernel-based techniques. Soft Computing. 2015;19(9):2469–2480. DOI: 10.1007/s00500-014-1573-5

[114] Wang S, Summers RM. Machine learning and radiology. Medical Image Analysis. 2012;16(5):933–951. DOI: 10.1016/j.media.2012.02.005

[115] De Nunzio G, Pastore G, Donativi M, Castellano A, Falini A. A CAD system for cerebral glioma based on texture features in DT-MR images. Nuclear Instruments and Methods in Physics Research Section A: Accelerators, Spectrometers, Detectors and Associated Equipment. 2011;648(1):S100–S102. DOI: 10.1016/j.nima.2010.12.086

[116] Tantisatirapong S, Nigel D, Rodriguez D, Abernethy L, Auer D, Clark C, et al. Magnetic resonance texture analysis: Optimal feature selection in classifying child brain tumors. In: XIII Mediterranean Conference on Medical and Biological Engineering and Com-

puting, MEDICON 2013, Springer, Sevilla, Spain; 2014. p. 309–312. DOI: 10.1007/978-3-319-00846-2_77

[117] Urish KL, Keffalas MG, Durkin JR, Miller DJ, Chu CR, Mosher TJ. T2 texture index of cartilage can predict early symptomatic OA progression: Data from the osteoarthritis initiative. Osteoarthritis and Cartilage. 2013;21(10):1550–1557. DOI: 10.1016/j.joca.2013.06.007

[118] Torheim T, Malinen E, Kvaal K, Lyng H, Indahl UG, Andersen EKF, Futsaether CM. Classification of dynamic contrast enhanced MR images of cervical cancers using texture analysis and support vector machines. IEEE Transactions on Medical Imaging. 2014;33(8):1648–1656. DOI: 10.1109/TMI.2014.2321024